Problem-Oriented Nursing Assessment

Problem-Oriented Nursing Assessment

PATRICIA DUBBERT LARKIN, M.A., R.N.
BARBARA A. BACKER, M.S., M.A., R.N.

Department of Nursing
Herbert H. Lehman College
of The City University of New York

McGRAW-HILL BOOK COMPANY

A Blakiston Publication

New York St. Louis San Francisco Auckland Bogotá
Düsseldorf Johannesburg London Madrid Mexico
Montreal New Delhi Panama Paris São Paulo
Singapore Sydney Tokyo Toronto

NOTICE

Medicine is an ever-changing science. As new research and clinical experience broaden our knowledge, changes in treatment and drug therapy are required. The editors and the publisher of this work have made every effort to ensure that the drug dosage schedules herein are accurate and in accord with the standards accepted at the time of publication. Readers are advised, however, to check the product information sheet included in the package of each drug they plan to administer to be certain that changes have not been made in the recommended dose or in the contraindications for administration. This recommendation is of particular importance in regard to new or infrequently used drugs.

Problem-Oriented Nursing Assessment

5 6 7 8 9 0 KPKP 8 3 2

This book was set in Univers by Allen Wayne Technical Corp.
The editor was Sally J. Barhydt;
the designer was Allen Wayne Technical Corp.;
the production supervisor was Milton J. Heiberg.
Kingsport Press was printer and binder.

Library of Congress Cataloging in Publication Data

Larkin, Patricia Dubbert.
Problem-oriented nursing assessment.

"A Blakiston publication."
Bibliography: p.
1. Nursing records. 2. Nursing. 3. Physical diagnosis. I. Backer, Barbara A., joint author. II. Title [DNLM: 1. Problem solving. 2. Nursing. WY100 L324p]
RT50.L37 610.73 76-41896
ISBN 0-07-036450-8

Contents

Preface

This text has been designed to help students carry out the nursing process using a collaborative approach with clients. It introduces students to problem solving, process recordings, and the problem-oriented health record. It also outlines a series of health status assessments. Obtaining the data for these health assessments provides a framework within which students can practice basic interviewing and technical skills. They learn to take health histories, perform beginning physical and mental health assessments, and analyze process recordings of selected interviews.

We believe that utilizing the nursing process, caring for clients as beginning primary care practitioners, should be the core of a first course in nursing. This is the time when students are forming their professional identities and assuming a new role; at this time they are also forming or re-forming their concept of what nursing really is. This workbook permits even beginning students to achieve a fairly complete and sophisticated assessment of the health status of their clients and guides them in identifying clients' strengths as well as problems that might require nursing intervention. In our nursing process course, students usually work with one client through the semester and are thus able to assume beginning-level responsibility and accountability for that client's nursing care. As teachers, we have been pleased with students' enthusiasm for this approach and their ability to use the data collected to formulate plans for working with clients, families, and other health professionals. Nurses already practicing and more experienced students may also find the workbook of value in that it presents a way of reviewing and implementing the nursing process while gaining familiarity with the problem-oriented system and examining interviewing skills.

This text is meant to be used along with—not instead of—textbook, classroom lecture and discussion, and audio-visual materials that present in depth the theoretical concepts that beginning students need as a foundation for their practice of nursing. Technical nursing care skills and physical assessment methods are not described here, but references are suggested for students who wish to review these.

Because we believe that the nurse-client relationship is such an integral part of the total nursing process, we have emphasized throughout the workbook the importance of listening to clients and working with them. Our presentation of the nursing process is based on the assumption that understanding interpersonal and problem-solving processes is fundamental to successful nursing practice.

Patricia Dubbert Larkin
Barbara A. Backer

Acknowledgments

We would like to express special thanks to:

Judith Rae Graves, whose unpublished paper on "The Nursing Process" and data collection outline preceded this text. She contributed to the development of the nursing process course and worked with us as a consultant in preparing the manuscript. Excerpts from her paper have been incorporated into the text on pages 1, 2, 3, 21, and 22.

Janet A. Rodgers, whose support and suggestions helped the idea for a workbook become a reality. She was the nursing process course coordinator during the time this text was being developed.

Claire Fagin, whose philosophy of nursing has inspired our thinking about what nursing is now and will be in the future.

Santa Pompei, for typing the manuscript for class use prior to publication.

Ira Bloom, for assisting us with permissions and arrangements for distributing the manuscript for class testing.

Barbara Starrett, for helping in preparing sample data.

Jewish Home and Hospital for Aged (Kingsbridge Center), for permission to use health record forms for sample data.

Armour Pharmaceuticals, for permission to use evaluation chart for activities of daily living.

Our colleagues, for suggestions and comments on the manuscript.

Parts of the assessment outline presented in this text are adapted from the Data Base Collection Outline developed by an ad hoc committee of the Herbert H. Lehman College Department of Nursing. Contributors to this committee included Shirlee Stokes, Patricia Larkin, Judith Graves, Judith Smith, Carolyn Ruda, Judy Lewis, and Elaine Eisenman.

The contents of Table 6-1, "Data Which May Be Collected in Each Assessment Area," in Pamela H. Mitchell, *Concepts Basic to Nursing,* McGraw-Hill, 1973, also suggested some parts of the assessment outline.

Finally, we wish to acknowledge and thank our students at Herbert H. Lehman College. Their enthusiasm for nursing and caring for clients are the best incentives to us as clinical instructors and we dedicate this text to them.

Patricia Dubbert Larkin
Barbara A. Backer

Problem-Oriented Nursing Assessment

UNIT 1

Introduction to Data Collection and Recording

OBJECTIVES

When you have completed this unit you should be able to:

1. State in your own words why nurses collect data and record their findings.
2. Define the following methods of collecting data:
   a. interviewing
   b. inspection
   c. palpation
   d. auscultation
   e. percussion
   f. consultation
3. Define and give examples of:
   a. subjective data
   b. objective data
4. Write an objective description of a person following the cephalocaudal approach.

PROBLEM SOLVING AND NURSING

It may surprise you to learn that your abilities as a professional nurse will depend to a considerable degree on your abilities as a problem solver. The reason is that, in our fast-changing world, the facts you learn in nursing school will not be enough ten years or even two years after you graduate. Without the ability to use problem solving, you would be forced to function by rote, uncreatively, depending on the facts you had memorized. Most likely, your knowledge would be obsolete soon after graduation. Although facts are important in nursing, the ability to put the facts together in a useful manner is what counts.

As you proceed through this workbook, you will be developing skills as a problem solver. You will be learning what facts are helpful, how to get information you need, and how to put the information together in a way that is helpful to you and to your clients. The *problem-oriented health record* (POHR) is a tool to help you with the process of problem solving in nursing. *Process recordings* are tools to help you analyze your interviewing skills and your relationship with a client.

NURSING ASSESSMENT

You may be wondering why nurses need all the assessment skills described in this workbook. Perhaps you thought it was the physician's role to assess a client's health status and that nurses merely obtained information from the physician. It is true that in many agencies a physician as well as a nurse assesses each client, and the information in the physician's history and physical examination is often every helpful to the nurse. However, the physician's assessment usually has a different focus or purpose than the nurse's. The physician collects data to identify and initiate medical intervention for health problems. The nurse collects data in order to identify and initiate intervention for problems that come within the scope of nursing. The following example concerning Mrs. MacGee, a client in her early thirties, indicates one way in which the nurse's and the physician's assessments may be complementary.

Mrs. MacGee came to the health care center because she had discovered a lump in her breast the previous week. In the initial interview and examination, the physician focused on diagnosing the disease process, and identified "lump in left breast" as a problem. The physician arranged for Mrs. MacGee to be admitted to the hospital for further tests. In keeping with the focus of nursing, the nurse's initial assessment concentrated on Mrs. MacGee's response to this change in her health status. The nurse determined that Mrs. MacGee was having difficulty making plans for leaving her two small children during the hospitalization. Review of the data also suggested to the nurse that Mrs. MacGee was very frightened of the surgical procedure and of the possibility of breast cancer. The nurse entered "child care during hospitalization" and "anxiety related to breast surgery" on Mrs. MacGee's problem list, and made plans to help Mrs. MacGee in these areas.

In many health care agencies, clients receive care from both nurses and physicians as well as from other health care professionals; and, as the above shows, each of these professionals requires data on which to base plans for helping the client. Obviously, whenever health care professionals are collaborating in the care of a client, it is important to avoid unnecessary duplication of effort in data gathering and problem solving. At times a client may depend on a nurse as his or her primary care practitioner. Then it is essential that the nurse be able to assess the client and determine his health care needs without relying on the expertise of other health care professionals, except when referral is indicated. The nurse will utilize the knowledge and skills of other health care practitioners and community resources when her assessment indicates the need.

Most people are familiar with physicians' assessments and treatments from their own or their families' experiences of acute illness. But what—more specifically than "helping sick people"—do they know of nursing assessment and intervention? The main goals of all nursing care are prevention of illness and maintenance or restoration of health. Nurses are concerned with helping clients cope with the practical problems of daily living brought about by their actual or potential health problems and with helping clients identify and utilize their strengths in dealing with these problems. The kind of information you need to be helpful as a professional nurse concerns the problems your client encounters in managing his daily living routines while coping with illness or disease, or trying to maintain or restore an optimum level of health. You and your clients will be using this information to work together to maximize their health capabilities. To get the information they need, nurses collect data about clients, their families, and their communities.

DATA COLLECTION

Collecting a data base is the first step of the nursing process and of all professional health assessment. The data, of course, are information. Data collected by professional nurses for their own practices will often also be of value to others in the health professions. It is important for you to recognize that this information gathering must be purposeful, discriminating, and systematic. Before you actually begin to collect data you must have a system to work with.

DATA SOURCES

Clients themselves are probably the richest source of data. The client's family also provides important data. Records may be another valuable source, particularly hospital and clinic charts. On such charts, you will find information recorded by other health professionals such as physicians, social workers, physical, occupational, and recreational therapists, pathologists, and laboratory technicians. At times you will also need to consult personally with other professionals to get information.

METHODS OF COLLECTING DATA

You receive information about your environment through your senses; the more senses you use and the better you use them, the more pertinent data you collect. Sometimes your senses will require mechanical assistance, but this will rarely be necessary. If you have not learned to use your own unaided senses with a high degree of competence, your skill in using mechanical aids will be of very little value.

Some very specific methods of data collection are used for health assessment. *Interviewing*, a way of talking with a client for a specific purpose, is the single most important method. A special form of interviewing known as "taking a history" has as its specific purpose the gathering of information about present or past health problems. You have already learned that the data you need as a nurse differ somewhat from what the physician needs, although there is some overlap. Accurate nursing diagnosis, like medical diagnosis, depends much more on a complete and accurate history than on a physical examination or clinical tests. Effective interviewing for any purpose depends upon the interviewer's skill in hearing what the client is saying by listening to his verbal language and by observing his facial expressions and body language. It also depends on the ability to create an environmental and interpersonal climate in which the client can relax and participate freely in the interview. In general, interviewing is most effective when the client feels free to talk about his problems as he sees them, and is encouraged to do so.

Inspection involves critical examination using the sense of vision. Observing the client is the first aspect of physical assessment. Observation is a difficult art to learn and requires that you be as objective as possible. Inspection is another major source of data. You will use it to look not only at people but also at books and records. Accuracy is vital, though difficult. Even talking with a client makes use of inspection because nonverbal messages are at least as important as the words actually spoken. The facial expression of a client, his body movements and position, his skin color and posture are all examples of observations that can be of significance to the client's health.

Auscultation, defined as the act of listening to assess health, generally implies listening by a mechanical aid such as a stethoscope. (The act of listening in nursing assessment is much broader, however, for we hear sighs and groans, cries and laughter, words and intonations that tell us about a person's health and feelings.)

Palpation means touching; in the context of nursing assessment, palpation refers to touching to gather data about temperature, texture, shape, size, motion, position, moisture, consistency, and tension. (You may also use palpation in the abstract sense, i.e., touching to convey caring.)

Percussion involves striking two bodies together to produce sound. In percussion of the human body, the sound emitted by tapping the surface with the examiner's fingers tells us about the density of underlying tissues. (Since percussion is not used in a beginning-level nursing assessment, it is not discussed further in this text.)

Consultation of records and other professionals has already been mentioned as an important data source.

THE CEPHALOCAUDAL APPROACH

Like all other data collection, physical examination is performed in a planned and organized way. It is helpful to look at the whole first, then the parts; when you begin the examination, write down your general impressions of clients as you first view them. This statement of general appearance should include the client's sex, approximate age, height and weight, posture and movements, dress, whether or not the client appears to be in acute discomfort, and any other characteristics that would single him or her out in a group. The accepted sequence of examination is to proceed (1) from the general, or the whole, to the specific, or the parts of the whole, (2) in a cephalocaudal ("head to tail") direction, and (3) from midline to periphery. You always begin an examination at the head and proceed downward and outward ending with the feet. Using this system will enable you to examine in a well-organized fashion without having to memorize a list of details to look for specifically.

SUBJECTIVE AND OBJECTIVE DATA

Accurate assessment requires the nurse to recognize the difference between subjective and objective data. *Subjective* data usually means the information obtained by interviewing the client, i.e., information about the client's health from his own point of view. A health history is composed of subjective data. It includes *symptoms* of illness identified by the client through his own self-awareness. Some very important data are purely subjective in nature—pain, for example. The client can tell the nurse about the location, timing, and characteristics of a pain, but it remains a personal experience and the nurse will never actually inspect, palpate, auscultate, or percuss the pain. Other examples of subjective data include a client's description of his home and family life, his report of past illnesses, his fears of having cancer, or his feelings of being nervous or depressed. The method used to gather subjective data is interviewing.

Objective data includes that which is observable and/or verifiable by clinical tests, *signs* of illness perceptible to someone other than the client alone. Grimacing, moaning, or clutching the chest are examples of objective data that might correspond to a client's subjective experience of chest pain. Other examples of objective data include skin rashes, body temperature, presence or absence of the knee jerk reflex, or a chest x-ray report. Inspection, palpation, auscultation, and percussion yield objective data. Laboratory test results are likewise objective data since they are scientifically verifiable.

The purpose of physical examination or laboratory testing is to provide objective data that will qualify and quantify the subjective data obtained through the health history interview. Therefore it is important that the summary of data collected from these examinations be presented in a way in which the results will not be biased by the subjective interpretations or judgments of the nurse. Note the difference in effect of the two descriptions given below.

Subjective description: "The client was very nervous."
Objective description: "The client spoke rapidly, crossed and uncrossed his legs several times, and drummed his fingers on the arm of the chair."

The latter objective description is far more accurate, especially since it is possible that the behaviors you might interpret as "nervousness" may be caused by something other than fear or anxiety. You may also wish to enhance the accuracy of your summary of the client's health history data by including exact quotations. Here are two acceptable ways of presenting subjective history data:

Example 1: Client states that the pain causes him to fear he may be having a "heart attack."
Example 2: Client states, "Whenever I feel that pain, I'm afraid I'm having a heart attack."

CONSULTING CLIENT CHARTS AND RECORDS

Each health care agency has developed a system for recording and preserving the records of health assessment and care provided for its clients. The contents of the client's chart or record vary with the purpose of the agency and with the number and kinds of health professionals involved in the client's care. A typical hospital chart will contain a history and physical examination, graphic sheets on which the client's temperature, pulse, respirations, and blood pressure are recorded at regular intervals, x-ray reports, laboratory test reports, and progress notes written by physicians, nurses, and other health practitioners. The traditional method of organizing the data in the chart was to enter all the reports of members of a given health profession in the same section. There would be separate sections, and perhaps color codes, for physicians' notes, nurses' notes, social workers' notes, laboratory reports, graphic sheets, and so on. Nurses have traditionally recorded nursing problems and nursing plans for intervention on the nursing Kardex. Many agencies still use this method of organizing client health care records.

The method you will be learning for nursing assessment is based on a newer way of organizing health records, which is described by Lawrence Weed and called the *problem-oriented* method. As the name implies, the problem-oriented method is organized around a list of health problems that are identified for each client. In this system, practitioners working with the client enter their notes sequentially, using the same basic format for writing up the information, and identifying by name and number the problem or problems to which the note applies. In some agencies in which the problem-oriented health record is used, nurses do not use the Kardex for recording nursing plans since these are already written in the client's record. The problem-oriented method of recording will be explained in more detail in succeeding units.

On the following pages are examples of the kind of data you might find in the chart of a woman recently admitted to a nursing home. The progress notes are more typical of those found in charts organized by the problem-oriented method. Note that the same information could be found in a traditional chart, but it would be organized in a different way. To help you interpret the records, we have preceded them with a list of abbreviations commonly used by health professionals.

ABBREVIATIONS COMMONLY USED IN HEALTH RECORDS

Ab.	abortion
a.c.	before food or meals
ad lib	to the amount desired
ADL	activities of daily living (eating, bathing, toileting, dressing, etc.)
ASA	acetylsalicylic acid (aspirin)
b.i.d.	twice a day
bm	bowel movement
BP	blood pressure
BRP	bathroom privileges (may get out of bed to use toilet)
Bx	biopsy
$\bar{c}$	with
Ca	cancer
CC	chief complaint
cc	cubic centimeter (equal to milliliter)
ct	client
dx	diagnosis, diagnostic
EEG	electroencephalogram
EKG or ECG	electrocardiogram
EENT	eye, ear, nose, throat
ER	emergency room
GI	gastrointestinal
gtt	drop, drops
GU	genitourinary
Gyn.	gynecological
h. or hr.	hour
h/o	history of
h.s.	hour of sleep (at bedtime)
hx	history
i or ṫ	one
I & O	intake and output
IM	intramuscular (injection)
IV	intravenous (injection or infusion)
L or Ⓛ or lt.	left
LE	lower extremity
ml	milliliter
MSE	mental status examination
neg	negative
nl	normal
noct.	at night
n.p.o.	nothing by mouth
Obs. or OB	obstetrics
o.d.	right eye
OPD	outpatient department
OR	operating room

o.s.	left eye
OT	occupational therapy
q.	every
q 2 hr.	every two hours
q.d.	every day
q.i.d.	four times a day
q.n.	every night
q.o.d.	every other day
q.s.	sufficient quantity
p.c.	after food or meals
PE	physical examination
Ped.	pediatrics
PERRLA	pupils equal, round, react to light and accommodation
PH	past (health) history
PI	present illness
p.o.	by mouth, orally
p.r.n.	as needed, when necessary
PT	physical therapy
PTA	prior to admission
R or Ⓡ or rt.	right
RBC	red blood cells
ROM	range of motion
RT	recreational therapy
Rx	therapy, therapeutic, treatment
s̄	without
sibs.	siblings
S.O.A.P.	subjective, objective, assessment, plan
SOB	shortness of breath
spec	specimen
stat	immediately
subcu. or subq.	subcutaneous (injection)
Sx	symptoms
t.i.d.	three times a day
TPR	temperature, pulse, and respirations
UE	upper extremity
VS	vital signs (temperature, pulse, respirations, blood pressure)
wnl	within normal limits
↑	increase, raise
↓	decrease, lower
ʒ	dram
℥	ounce
♀	female
♂	male
⟶	to, toward
>	greater than
<	less than

FIGURE 1-1. SAMPLE PROGRESS RECORD

THE JEWISH HOME AND HOSPITAL FOR AGED

KINGSBRIDGE CENTER

PROGRESS RECORD

Smith, Mary
Rm. 506A

Instructions: A red line is drawn across the sheet after each day's notes.

DATE AND TIME	NURSING NOTES	DATE	MEDICAL NOTES
		6/5/75	#2 Pain in Knees + ankles.
			S. Pt. c/o AM stiffness on
			arising - gets better but later
			on in day easy fatiguability.
			Pt. denies swelling or redness.
			Also has some proximal inter-
			phalangeal stiffness. Pt. states
6/7/75	#2 Pain in Knees and ankles		H/O rheumatoid arthritis
10 A.M.	S. Ct. states hot packs in P.T.		relieved by acetylsalicylic
	"really helped", relieved pain.		acid, P.T., and heat.
	"It's easier for me to walk".		O. UE: hands - no swelling,
	O. Swelling still noticeable in		no atrophy, full ROM.
	both Knees. Able to walk c̄ walker		LE: Knees - bilateral
	around room. Taking acetylsalicylic		swelling, tenderness to
	acid as prescribed. Naps for hr. in		palpation and active ROM,
	AM and p̄ lunch. Maintains self care		no limitation in ROM.
	in ADL.		ankles - ō swelling,
	A. Acetylsalicylic acid and hot		full ROM, ō tenderness.
	packs in P.T. relieving pain.		A. Arthritis, probably
	P. Dx- (1) evaluate exercise tolerance.		rheumatoid according to HX.
	(2) monitor side effects of		P. DX - sed rate, latex
	acetylsalicylic acid.		RX - (1) acetylsalicylic
	Rx- (1) continue acetylsalicylic		acid, 600 mg p.o. q 4 hr.
	acid p.o. q4 hrs prn		prn pain.
	and hot packs q d.		(2) to go to P.T.
	(2) support self-care by non-		S. Bardo, M.D.
	hurried approach 1. plan c̄ ct.		
	best time for bathing, activities		
	2. plan rest periods, especially p̄		
	shower q.o.d		
	(3) ambulate c̄ walker		
	Teaching-(1) moving from walker to		

FIGURE 1-1. SAMPLE PROGRESS RECORD (cont.)

THE JEWISH HOME AND HOSPITAL FOR AGED

KINGSBRIDGE CENTER

PROGRESS RECORD

Instructions: A red line is drawn across the sheet after each day's notes.

Smith, Mary
Rm. 506 A

DATE AND TIME	NURSING NOTES	DATE	MEDICAL NOTES
	chair and back.		
	(2) use of hand rails in B.R.		
	Referral - (1) confer ē P.T. re ct's		
	progress on unit.		
	M. Alexander, R.N.		
6/8/75	#3 Fear of falling		
	S. "The pain is better but I		
	don't like that walker."		
	O. Sitting most of day. Related		
	fear of falling to daughter during		
	visit this A.M. Daughter says ct		
	used walker once before and fell		
	ē injury.		
	A. Ct fears falling ē walker.		
	Continued mobility important for		
	ROM and self-esteem.		
	P. Dx - (1) Discuss ē ct. feelings		
	Rx - about use of walker,		
	ambulation, other concerns.		
	(2) check safety conditions in		
	room - clean, dry floor, furniture		
	spaced, + cords, wires, out of way.		
	Teaching - (1) review teaching		
	safe use of walker, remain ē		
	ct during transfers.		
	Referral - (1) Confer ē P.T. re:		
	possible alternatives to walker.		
	M. Alexander, R.N.		
6/8/75	#4 ↓ Appetite		
7:30 pm	S. States "I can't eat"		
	O. Refused dinner, eating very		
	little @ other meals today		

FIGURE 1-1. SAMPLE PROGRESS RECORD (cont.)

THE JEWISH HOME AND HOSPITAL FOR AGED

KINGSBRIDGE CENTER

PROGRESS RECORD

Smith, Mary
Rm. 506 A

Instructions: A red line is drawn across the sheet after each day's notes.

DATE AND TIME	NURSING NOTES	DATE	MEDICAL NOTES
6/8/75 cont.	A. ↓ appetite. May be developing gastric irritation from ASA, worried about something, or may have food preferences not being acknowledged. P. Dx: 1) discuss food likes and dislikes, 2) initiate I+O record, Rx: 1) allow time daily for ct to discuss concerns, 2) give ASA with milk or snack, Teaching: deferred until problem clarified. Dx - add: check V.S. q.d. R. Brown, R.N.		

FIGURE 1-2. GRAPHIC SHEET

THE JEWISH HOME AND HOSPITAL FOR AGED
KINGSBRIDGE CENTER

GRAPHIC SHEET

Smith, Mary
Rm. 506A

Date	Hour	Temp.	Pulse	Resp.	B/P	Weight	Bath	Stool	Urine	Intravenous	Intake 24 Hr.	Output 24 Hr.	Misc.
6/1/75	8PM						Shower	Ṫ	BRP				
6/2/75	8PM	37.0	72	16	150/90			Ṫ	BRP				
6/3/75	8PM						Shower	Ṫ	BRP				
6/4/75	8PM	37.0	70	18	146/90			Ṫ	BRP				
6/5/75	8PM						Shower		BRP				
6/6/75	8PM	37.0	74	18	150/90			Ṫ	BRP				
6/7/75	8PM						Shower		BRP				
6/8/75	8PM	37.7	82	22	154/90		Bedbath				100cc	175cc	→ (started at 6PM. 6/8/75)
6/9/75	8PM	37.6	90	20	150/88						600cc	750cc	
6/10/75	8PM	37.0	76	18	140/90		Shower	Ṫ			1200cc	860cc	
6/11/75	8PM	36.8	68	16	144/86			Ṫ			2000cc	1180cc	

Form 109 — Apollo

FIGURE 1-3. BLOOD CHEMISTRY, HEMATOLOGY, URINALYSIS

THE JEWISH HOME AND HOSPITAL FOR AGED

BLOOD CHEMISTRY

NAME Smith, Mary ROOM 506A DATE 6/1/75 DR. Bard

Test	Result	Unit	Test	Result	Unit	Test	Result	Unit
☒ SUGAR	192	mg %	☒ SODIUM	143	meq	☐ AMYLASE		units
☐ UREA N		mg %	☒ POTASSIUM	4.8	meq	☐ SGOT		units per m
☐ CREATININE		mg %	☒ CHLORIDES	107	meq	☐ LACTIC DEHYDR.		units
☐ URIC ACID		mg %	☒ CO_2	24 meq	val %	☐ P B I		mcgm/100 ml
☐ CALCIUM		mg %	☐ BILIRUBIN		mg %	GLUCOSE TOLERANCE		
☒ TOTAL PROTEIN	6.0	%	☐ PROTHROMBIN		sec.	☐ FASTING		mg %
☐ ALBUMIN		%	☐ CONTROL		sec.	☐ ½ Hr.		mg %
☐ GLOBULIN		%	☐ CEPH. FLOCC.		24 hr.	☐ 1 Hr.		mg %
☐ IN. PHOSPHORUS		mg %	☐ THYMOL TURB.		units	☐ 2 Hrs.		mg %
☐ ALK. PHOSPH.		SJR units	☐ CHOLESTEROL		mg %	☐ 3 Hrs.		mg %
☐ ACID PHOSPH.		SJR units	☐ CHOL. ESTERS		mg %	☐		

THE JEWISH HOME AND HOSPITAL FOR AGED

HEMATOLOGY

NAME Smith, Mary ROOM 506A DATE 6/1/75 DR. Bard

	DIFFERENTIAL	
HGB 9.6		BL. TIME ______ min.
RBC 4.3 x 10^6	POLYS ______	CL. TIME ______ min.
WBC 6,000	BANDS ______	PLATELETS ______
	LYMPH ______	RETICULOCYTE ______ %
ESR ______ mm/h	MONO ______	REMARKS ______
	EOS ______	
HEMATOCRIT 30.1 mm	BASO ______	

THE JEWISH HOME AND HOSPITAL FOR AGED

URINALYSIS

NAME Smith, Mary ROOM 506A DATE 6/1/75 DR. Bard

	MICROSCOPIC	STOOL ANALYSIS
SP. GR. 1.011		
REACT. ALK. NEUT. ACID ______	EPITH. ______	BLOOD 0
COLOR gold amber	R B C ______	
ALBUMIN ______	W B C clumps	
SUGAR neg	CASTS ______	
ACETONE neg	BACTERIA ______	
BILE ______	OTHER ______	
UROBILINOGEN ______		

FIGURE 1-4. MEDICATION RECORD

MEDICATION RECORD
STAT, PRN and I.V. MEDICATIONS

1. Record Stat, PRN and I.V. Medications on this form.
2. Use Blue Medication Record for standing orders.
3. If a medication is refused or not given, record an explanation on the Nurses' Note Sheet.
4. Record pulse rate in v.s. (vital signs) column when cardiotonics are given.
5. Sign full name and initials once on back of Medication record.

THE JEWISH HOME AND HOSPITAL FOR AGED
Kingsbridge Center

Allergic To: PENICILLIN
(Record in Red)

Smith, Mary
506 A

Date	MEDICATIONS	TIME	V.S	Initial	Date	MEDICATIONS	TIME	V.S	Initial	Date	MEDICATIONS	TIME	V.S	Initial
6/5/75	Acetylsalicylic Acid 600 mg po q 4hr prn	8		mm										
		3		mm										
		9		RB										
6/6/75	Acetylsalicylic Acid 600 mg po q 4hr prn	6		KP										
		11		mm										
		5		RB										
6/7/75	Acetylsalicylic Acid 600 mg po q 4hr prn	8		mm										
		12		mm										
		5		RB										
		9		RB										
6/8/75	Acetylsalicylic Acid 600 mg po q 4hr prn	11		mm										
		6		RB										
		10		RB										
6/9/75	Acetylsalicylic Acid 600 mg po q 4hr prn	1		CS										
		8		mm										
		5		RB										
	Milk of Magnesia 30 cc po	10		RB										

FIGURE 1-5. KARDEX

882 - RRNT-36006A

ORDER DATE	REORDER DATE	MEDICATIONS	STOP DATE
6/1/75		Milk of Magnesia 30 cc po qod prn constipation 10 PM	
6/5/75		Acetylsalicylic Acid 600 mg po q4hr prn	

ACTIVITIES OF DAILY LIVING — ACTIVITIES OF DAILY LIVING

882 - RRNT-37448 C

ACTIVITIES
- [ ] BEDREST
- [ ] DANGLE
- [ ] CHAIR
- [ ] WHEELCHAIR
- [x] WALKER
- [ ] UP AD LIB

SIDE RAILS
- [ ] CONSTANTLY
- [x] NIGHTS ONLY
- [ ] BOTH
- [ ] ONE

HYGIENE
- [ ] BED BATH
- [ ] PARTIAL BATH
- [ ] SELF BATH
- [ ] TUB
- [x] SHOWER in chair c̄ help

ALLERGIES (IN RED)

Penicillin

DIET
- [x] REGULAR
- [ ] OTHER (SPECIFY)

FEEDING
- [x] SELF
- [ ] ASSIST

MENTAL STATUS
- [x] ALERT
- [ ] CHEERFUL
- [ ] DEPRESSED
- [ ] DISORIENTED

ORIENTATION TO MEMORY
- [x] GOOD
- [ ] FAIR
- [ ] POOR
- [ ] OTHER (SPECIFY)

BOWEL / BLADDER
- [ ] COLOSTOMY
- [ ] INCONTINENT
- [ ] CATHETER
- [ ] BEDPAN / URINAL
- [ ] COMMODE
- [x] B R P c̄ help
- [ ] INTAKE
- [ ] OUTPUT
- [ ] CLINITEST
- [ ] BOWEL / BLADDER
- [ ] TRAINING
- [ ] OTHER

VITAL SIGNS
- [ ] O D
- [ ] B I D
- [ ] T I D
- [ ] OTHER

Routine

APPLIANCES
- [ ] EYEGLASSES
- [x] HEARING AID
- [ ] PACEMAKER

PHYSICAL TRAITS
- [ ] LEFT HANDED
- [x] RIGHT HANDED
- [ ] PARAPLEGIC
- [ ] HEMIPLEGIC L____ R____
- [ ] BLIND L____ R____
- [ ] DEAF L____ R____
- [ ] SPEECH IMPEDIMENT
- [ ] OTHER (SPECIFY)

THERAPY
- [ ] O. T.
- [x] P. T.
- [ ] R. T.
- [ ] OTHER

PROSTHESIS
- [ ] DENTURES
- [ ] EYE
- [ ] LIMB
- [ ] OTHER (SPECIFY)

NAME MARY SMITH ROOM 506 A

BIBLIOGRAPHY

If you are learning or need to review the basic interviewing and technical nursing skills needed to carry out the assessments described in this workbook, you may find the list of suggested readings helpful. Audio-visual materials are also available and some suggestions are included in Appendix 1. The references listed are not meant to be inclusive, but are seen by the authors as providing a theoretical framework for the assessment content. Some of the references describe how to perform the basic nursing skills necessary to complete the assessments. Others provide assessment techniques that are more advanced and sophisticated than the beginning-level assessments described in this text. These sources will be helpful to you if you wish to expand your skills and data base in some of the assessment areas.

SELECTED BIBLIOGRAPHY

Nursing and Changing Roles

Mauksch, Ingeborg G.: "Nursing Is Coming of Age . . . through the Practitioner Movement," *American Journal of Nursing,* **75**:1834-1843, 1975.

Mitchell, Pamela Holsclaw: *Concepts Basic to Nursing,* McGraw-Hill, New York, 1977, pp. 25-31.

Problem Solving in Nursing

Fuerst, Elinor V., LuVerne Wolff, and Marlene H. Weitzel: *Fundamentals of Nursing,* 5th ed., J.B. Lippincott, Philadelphia, 1975, pp. 55-62.

Marriner, Ann: *The Nursing Process,* C.V. Mosby, St. Louis, 1975, pp. 1-4.

Mitchell, Pamela Holsclaw: *Concepts Basic to Nursing,* McGraw-Hill, New York, 1977, pp. 52-57.

Communication of Health Status Data

Fuerst, Elinor V., LuVerne Wolff, and Marlene H. Weitzel: *Fundamentals of Nursing,* 5th ed., J.B. Lippincott, Philadelphia, 1975, pp. 93-98.

Assessment Skills

Alexander, Mary M., and Marie Scott Brown: "Physical Examination, Part 1, The How and Why of Examination," *Nursing '73,* **3**:25-28, July 1973.

Bates, Barbara: *Physical Examination,* J.B. Lippincott, Philadelphia, 1974, pp. 5-7.

Mitchell, Pamela Holsclaw: *Concepts Basic to Nursing,* McGraw-Hill, New York, 1977, pp. 83-85, 97-104.

The Problem-Oriented Record

Weed, Lawrence: "Medical Records That Guide and Teach," *New England Journal of Medicine,* **278**:593-600, March 1968.

DATE:

ASSESSMENT PRACTICE 1: Objective Description

Now you are ready to begin using some of the data collection methods described in the previous pages. To complete the exercises in this workbook it is usually not necessary to practice with a person actually identified as a client in a health service agency. You can learn the skills by practicing with a classmate, friend, or other willing subject as long as someone qualified to supervise and validate your work is available during the learning process. It is highly recommended that you always practice the skills as through you were in a real clinical situation and that you actually perform the assessments with identified clients as soon as possible after gaining competency in each assessment area.

As you perform the assessments described in this workbook, you will be learning some of the skills that are necessary for a complete physical and mental health examination. To sharpen your ability to observe and describe accurately and objectively, write out a description of a person. Follow the general-to-specific, cephalocaudal, midline-to-periphery approach and use objective terms. Practice the skill of inspection.

General appearance:

Head:

Hair:

Eyes:

Eyebrows:

Ears:

Nose:

Mouth:

Neck:

Chest:

Arms:

Hands:

Abdomen:

Legs:

Feet:

Emotional expression:

DATE:

ASSESSMENT PRACTICE 2: Subjective and Objective Data

Classify the sample data according to whether they are subjective or objective. What data collection methods were probably used to collect the data?

	Subjective	Objective	Data Collection Methods
Constipation			
Pain in legs	X		interviewing
Pulse			
Number of stools			
Fear of falling			
Red blood count			
Food likes and dislikes			
Respirations		X	palpation, inspection, auscultation
Joint stiffness			
Urine specific gravity			

UNIT 2

Interpreting Data and Identifying Problems

OBJECTIVES

When you have completed this unit you should be able to:

1. Interpret data from sample health record data.
2. Compare data in the sample records to norms.
3. Identify actual or potential problems and strengths from the sample data.
4. Formulate client-identified problems from the sample data.
5. Begin a problem list based on the sample data.

INTERPRETING DATA

The next step in problem solving, after careful data collection, is interpretation and analysis of the data. The data collected by a professional nurse concern health, and the information is used to identify the client's health status and evaluate the effectiveness of care. Some data are relatively easy to interpret by comparing with norms listed in tables, for example, height, weight, chemical blood values, and vital signs. Other data—e.g., child rearing practices or emotional responses—require more skill to interpret.

Before you begin interpreting the sample data in the previous unit, let us review the concept of "normal." Normal means average or most usual. Physical and laboratory norms are determined by measuring a specific quantity on a large number of subjects chosen at random. The values of most subjects will fall within a certain range around the average. A normal adult heart rate, for example, may be anywhere between 60 and 100 beats per minute, but most adults have a heart rate between 72 and 80 beats per minute. Values less than 60 and more than 100 are frequently but not always associated with physical or emotional states that are not considered healthy.

Normal also varies with factors such as age, sex, and socioeconomic and ethnic background. A 6-foot adult male is not considered abnormally tall in the United States, but a 6-foot adult woman or ten-year-old boy would be unusual. So, by comparing the data with appropriate norms for the client in terms of age, sex, or other appropriate criteria, you can decide whether the data fall within or outside the normal range.

What do you do to determine whether or not a given behavior is normal? You can't measure factors such as irritability, activity, or child-rearing practices as easily or objectively as blood pressure. Norms in these instances depend heavily on culture and the mores set by society. Thus, before interpreting many behaviors, you must evaluate them in view of the expectations and values of the client's culture or subculture. Behavior different from what is expected in light of culture may well indicate a deviation from normal for an individual. Often you must know an individual fairly well before you can accurately interpret behavior. All behavior has meaning, and until you can determine with the client what significance a particular behavior has for her or him, you cannot accurately interpret it.

IDENTIFYING AND LISTING PROBLEMS

You already know that the object of collecting and interpreting health status data is for the nurse to determine the client's problems, strengths, and ways of coping. In beginning assessment, whenever you find data to be outside the normal range, you should consider this a problem until you know otherwise. In general, problems fall into one of five categories:

1. Anything that is unusual and not explained, and requires further investigation or verification.
   Example: unexplained weight loss or gain
2. Anything that is unusual and is explained, but requires professional attention.
   Example: allergy to penicillin
3. Anything the client considers a problem.
   Examples: fear of elevators, no health clinic within easy commuting distance
4. Potential or high-risk problems secondary to client's age, sex, history, or ethnicity
   Examples: cataracts, sickle cell anemia, birth defects, genetic diseases, black lung disease
5. Health maintenance. Although deviations from normal health may be easier to identify, helping a client to recognize and mobilize his strengths in order to maintain health or cope with problems is probably one of the most important functions of professional nursing. Health maintenance activities by nurse and client are necessary whenever specific strengths or levels of "wellness" may be lost or diminished without frequent attention.
   Examples: immunizations against contagious diseases, regular dental and eye examinations, brushing teeth after meals, maintaining skin cleanliness, and performing range of joint motion exercises

When you list a problem, always include the following:

1. The *date* when the problem was identified by the practitioner. (Note that in some agencies, the date of onset of the problem is listed instead of or in addition to the date when the problem was identified.)
2. The *name* of the problem in terms of the level at which you understand it. This means that if the graphic sheet indicates a pulse rate ranging from 104 to 120 beats per minute, you would list the problem as "pulse consistently greater than 100," not "heart disease." Do not make diagnostic guesses.

Examples:

#1	8/14/72	Allergic to diazepam (Valium)
#2	8/20/72	Temperature elevation
#3	8/22/72	Family does not visit (client-identified problem)
#4	8/25/72	History of suicide attempts
#5	8/25/72	Maintain participation in weight loss club

As you see, problems may be medical, psychological, social, or demographic.

SELECTED BIBLIOGRAPHY

Evaluating and Interpreting Data

Durand, Mary, and Rosemary Prince: "Nursing Diagnosis: Process and Decision," *Nursing Forum,* 5 (4):50-64, 1966. Also reprinted in Ann Marriner, *The Nursing Process,* C. V. Mosby, St. Louis, 1975, pp. 60-68.

Fuerst, Elinor V., LuVerne Wolff, and Marlene H. Weitzel: *Fundamentals of Nursing,* 5th ed., J. B. Lippincott, Philadelphia, 1974, pp. 63-71.

Mitchell, Pamela Holsclaw: *Concepts Basic to Nursing,* McGraw-Hill, New York, 1977, pp. 106–116.

DATE:

ASSESSMENT PRACTICE 3: Interpreting Data

Compare the data in the sample client records found in Unit 1 to norms. You can find normal values in nursing, medical, anatomy and physiology, and pharmacology textbooks. Use the data collection method of consultation and the problem-solving skill of interpretation.

	Client Data	Norms
Temperature		
Pulse		
Blood pressure		diastolic 60-90mm Hg* systolic 95-140mm Hg*
24-h fluid intake		
Stools		3 per day to 1 per week†
Urine color		
Urine specific gravity		
Hemoglobin		
Hemotocrit		
White blood count		
Respirations		
Dosage of aspirin		
Dosage of milk of magnesia		
Urine sugar		
Urine acetone		
Blood sugar		
Serum sodium		
Serum potassium		

*Carol Gilbert, "Physical Appraisal of Circulatory Function," in Josephine M. Sana and Richard D. Judge (eds.), *Physical Appraisal Methods in Nursing Practice,* Little, Brown, Boston, 1975, p. 191.
†Pamela Holsclaw Mitchell, *Concepts Basic to Nursing,* McGraw-Hill, New York, 1977, p. 367.
Note: Lab values may vary among agencies depending on techniques used.

DATE:

ASSESSMENT PRACTICE 4: Identifying Problems

Problem List: Identify problems from the sample data in Unit 1. Include one or more from the categories of actual and potential and client-identified problems. List these below. (Try to identify problems not already specified in the progress notes.)

Problem Number	Date Identified	Problem Name	Date Resolved/Inactive

Client Strengths and Health Maintenance: Identify at least one strength or area of health to be maintained from the sample data.

UNIT 3

Interviewing and Use of Process Recordings

OBJECTIVES

When you have completed this unit you should be able to:

1. Explain the purpose of participant observation in interacting with clients.
2. State the purpose(s) and goal(s) of your interview with a client.
3. State your preconceptions about your client and the interview.
4. Record and interpret the verbal and nonverbal responses that occurred between you and the client during the interview.
5. Evaluate the effectiveness of your interaction with the client.

INTERVIEWING

Communication skills are vital to nursing problem solving: interviewing, as you will recall from Unit 1, is the most important tool of data collection. Interviewing may have different goals and purposes, and the practitioner utilizes various techniques to meet these different objectives. For example, in utilizing the interviewing form of history taking for the stated goal of finding out what and how the client reports about his health status, you will be asking your client some direct and specific questions. However, as you ask these questions, you may note that the client digresses at times from a specific question to talk about something else that is of concern to him. You may need to help the client refocus on the specific topic being discussed, or you may decide that what the client is introducing as a topic of concern is important to discuss at that time. It is important to have a goal for your interview in order to provide direction for your and the client's participation, and to help you set priorities. Other factors involved in determining priorities are the degree of discomfort the client may be experiencing, the immediate need for specific information and/or intervention, and the amount of time you may have to spend with the client. Goals for other forms of interviewing may be to listen, to talk with the client about what is of concern to him, and to help him recognize, utilize, and develop his own strengths in understanding situations and problems and in coping with them. How comfortable the nurse and the client feel in the interview situation and how much trust has developed in their relationship will influence what is or is not said.

While the client and nurse are engaged in the interview, it is possible for the nurse to collect data about both participants and the interaction between them. The process by which you, the nurse, participate in the interaction with the client and at the same time observe the relationship between the client and yourself is called *participant observation.* This process is a very helpful tool in nursing, because you are looking at the behavior and responses of both yourself and the client with the purpose of understanding these and perhaps other interactions that may be related. Through participant observation, the nurse can review the strengths and weaknesses of both participants.

PROCESS RECORDINGS

Analyzing your own participant observation with clients is one way to learn effective interviewing techniques. To do this you need an accurate record or description of the interaction. The most accurate record would be a film or videotape that would document verbal and nonverbal behavior. Tape recordings and notes on the dialogue written during the interview rank next best, while a description based on what the interviewer recalls after the interview ends is the least complete and least accurate. How you record the interaction will depend on the equipment available, agency restrictions, and the kind of relationship you have with a client.

Process recordings are written descriptions by the practitioner of the verbal and nonverbal responses of nurse and client occurring during the interaction and recorded either during the interview or afterwards. Process recordings usually consist of two parts: (1) a verbatim recording and description of the verbal and nonverbal behavior during the interaction, and (2) an analysis or interpretation of the meaning and significance of the recorded behavior.

HOW TO WRITE A PROCESS RECORDING

As a participant observer in an interview, and when writing a process recording, it is helpful to follow these steps:

1. Note the date, time, place, and any significant environmental features (lighting, other persons in the area, nearby activity, or other distractions).
2. State your long-term and immediate goals.
3. Write a brief general description (refer to Unit 1) of the client as he or she appeared before the interview began.
4. Briefly describe your own preconceptions about the client, the interview situation, and your own behavior at the time just before the interview.
5. Write down the interaction as it actually occurred; record exactly what the client said and did and exactly what you said, what you thought and felt, and what you did. This is your observation of your own behavior as you participate in the relationship.
6. Read over the entire interaction. You are now ready to interpret and evaluate your interview.
7. Identify the *content* (what was said, done). Try to pick out a theme or themes (examples: loneliness, worry over family).
8. Identify the mood or moods (the feeling-tone)(examples: anger, joy, sadness).
9. Try to identify the *process.* How were you and the client stimulating and responding to each other's behavior? (examples: moving closer, developing trust, creating distance, testing each other).
10. Notice where content and/or moods change. Try to determine what was happening at that time and why (examples: silences develop, one of you becomes more anxious, the subject is changed).

11. Review your responses to the client. Which were effective communication techniques and which were ineffective? Were the participants receiving each other's messages?
12. Evaluate the interaction as a whole. What did you learn? What did the client learn? Were your goals accomplished?

Review of your process recording may help you to identify your client's strengths as well as new areas of concern that you may decide to add to your problem list. Although they are not part of the problem-oriented health record, process recordings will help you solve problems in the areas of communications and interpersonal relationships. Several process recordings documenting a series of interviews with the same client can be especially helpful in learning about the development and changes in a professional relationship over time. Nursing students are usually required to review their process recordings with instructors, but graduate nurses may ask peers or clinical specialists in psychiatric and mental health nursing to help them analyze the interactions they have recorded. Sometimes the analysis and interpretation is written and sometimes it consists of a discussion between the nurse and the person assisting the nurse to understand its meaning. Asking another practitioner to review the interaction data is helpful because it is often difficult to look objectively at one's own behavior.

It is helpful to remember as you review your process recording that what happened in the interaction needs to be looked at not in terms of "right" or "wrong," but in terms of "What can I learn from this? What did I respond to and help the client with, or what did I miss? If I did miss a cue or comment, what was happening at this point in the interaction so I can learn from this and perhaps next time be more aware of this?" Participant observation and process recordings are tools with which you may learn about yourself and how you use nursing theory. They will also help you learn about, and help, your clients. You may wish to use sources in the Unit 3 bibliography or other references to help you interpret and evaluate your interaction and improve your interviewing skills.

Parts of one process recording are shown in the following example.

PROCESS RECORDING

Date	6/7/75	**Client**	Mrs. R., age 82
Nurse	Carol Briggs	**Time**	1 P.M.
Place	Fairview Nursing Home		

Significant Environmental Factors
Well-lit, comfortably furnished private room. No other people present.

Long-term Goals
To help Mrs. R. maintain optimum health status, considering her age and her strengths, and to establish a trusting relationship between the two of us.

Short-term Goals

To initiate relationship and to listen to what Mrs. R. introduces as topics of concern.

Description of Client

Mrs. R. a small, thin, elderly woman about 5 feet tall and appearing her stated age was sitting on the bed in her room. Her posture was stiff and straight, her skin color was pale, and her hands were folded in her lap. She was dressed in a navy blue suit, white blouse, and navy shoes. Her grey hair was combed into a bun. She wore glasses and no makeup. She had no expression on her face and she was looking at the wall.

Preconceptions

I wasn't very sure of what I was going to say to Mrs. R. about what our relationship was going to be. I wished I had had more experience as a nurse! I thought that because of the difference in our ages Mrs. R. and I wouldn't have anything to talk about. She reminded me of my grandmother.

Client Behavior and Response	Nurse Behavior and Response	Interpretations and Conclusions
	I walked into the room and said, "Good afternoon, Mrs. R., my name is Carol Briggs." I wondered if Mrs. R. would talk to me at all. She was always alone when I passed her room. I stood to the side of the bed and had my hands in my uniform pocket. My fists were clenched and my mouth felt very dry.	
"Good afternoon," Mrs. R. smiled. "Are you a nurse?"	"Yes well, not exactly. I'm a student nurse at the college and I'm here every Monday."	I felt relief that Mrs. R. had answered me. I didn't know what I was going to do or say if she hadn't responded.
"That's nice. This is a nice home. I've been here 13 months. I get along as best I can but its so hard sometimes. . . ."	"Its hard. . . .?"	I wanted to encourage Mrs. R. to talk more about what she thought was hard for her. Peplau states that nurses can help a client to learn about a difficulty by encouraging him to describe it.* I also did not know what Mrs. R. really meant by that.

*Hildegard E. Peplau, "Professional Closeness," *Nursing Forum,* **69**:349, 1969.

PROCESS RECORDING (cont.)

Client Behavior and Response	Nurse Behavior and Response	Interpretation and Conclusions
"Would you like to see the scarf I'm knitting?" Mrs. R. went to her bureau drawer and took out a scarf.	I smiled. "It looks lovely."	Although I didn't think of it at the time, I see now that Mrs. R. changed the subject as I tried to help her talk about her feelings.
Mrs. R. smiled. "Do you really think so?"	"Yes, I like it."	I was happy that my opinion was important to her.
Silence Mrs. R. kept looking at me.	Silence	I didn't know where to go from here and I felt very uncomfortable. My preconception that Mrs. R. and I wouldn't have anything to talk about seemed to be coming true!
	"May I sit down and talk with you for a few minutes?"	
"Please do. It's so nice to have a young person like you to stop in and talk. No one here seems to have time to pay any attention to me."	I sat down in the chair next to Mrs. R.'s bed.	Both Mrs. R. and I seemed to relax at this point. Mrs. R. started to talk a bit more about her feelings. I think my stating my goal a little more clearly helped to decrease both her anxiety and mine! Both of us now were sitting down, which also seemed to create a more comfortable climate for talking.

SELECTED BIBLIOGRAPHY

Communication Skills in Nursing

Becknell, Eileen Pearlman, and Dorothy M. Smith: *System of Nursing Practice,* F. A. Davis, Philadelphia, 1975, pp. 35-39.

Fuerst, Elinor V., LuVerne Wolff, and Marlene H. Weitzel: *Fundamentals of Nursing,* 5th ed, J. B. Lippincott, Philadelphia, 1974, pp. 101-108, 119-128.

Goldin, Phyllis, and Barbara Russell: "Therapeutic Communication," *American Journal of Nursing,* **69:**1928-1930, 1969. Also reprinted in Ann Marriner, *The Nursing Process,* C. V. Mosby, St. Louis, 1975, pp. 166-169.

Hays, Joyce S., and Kenneth H. Larson: *Interacting with Patients,* Macmillan, New York, 1974.

Hewitt, Helen E., and Betty L. Pesznecker: "Blocks To Communicating with Patients," *American Journal of Nursing,* **64:**101-103, July 1964. Also reprinted in Ann Marriner, *The Nursing Process,* C. V. Mosby, St. Louis, 1975, pp. 170-174.

Marriner, Ann: *The Nursing Process,* C. V. Mosby, St. Louis, 1975, pp. 21-24.

Marsden, Alice, and Josephine M. Sana: "Nurse-Patient Communication and Relationship in the Physical Appraisal Process," in Josephine M. Sana and Richard D. Judge (eds.), *Physical Appraisal Methods in Nursing Practice,* Little, Brown, Boston, 1975, pp. 65-78.

Mercer, Lianne S., and Patricia O'Connor: *Fundamental Skills in the Nurse-Patient Relationship,* W. B. Saunders, Philadelphia, 1974.

Mitchell, Pamela Holsclaw: *Concepts Basic to Nursing,* McGraw-Hill, New York, 1977, pp. 58–79, 85–97.

Orlando, Ida: *The Dynamic Nurse-Patient Relationship,* G.P. Putnam's Sons, New York, 1961.

Peplau, Hildegard E.: *Interpersonal Relations in Nursing,* G. P. Putnam's Sons, New York, 1952.

_____ "Professional Closeness," *Nursing Forum,* **69:**342-360, 1969.

_____ "Talking with Patients," *American Journal of Nursing,* **60** (7):964-966, 1960. Also reprinted in Ann Marriner, *The Nursing Process,* C.V. Mosby, St. Louis, 1975, pp. 161-165.

Travelbee, Joyce: *Interpersonal Aspects of Nursing,* F. A. Davis, Philadelphia, 1966.

Ujhely, Gertrude: *Determinants of the Nurse-Patient Relationship,* Springer Publishing, New York, 1968.

DATE:

ASSESSMENT PRACTICE 5: Process Recording

Plan to interview a client. Before the interview, decide on your goals for the interaction. As soon as possible after the interview, write a process recording of your interaction with the client. Follow the steps outlined in this unit. It is helpful to record at least fifteen minutes of the dialogue in the interview. You may not be able to remember all that happened, but try to record sequentially exactly what was said and done. After you have written the process recording, plan to review it with your instructor. Since you were a participant observer in the interaction, a third person may provide objective observations which you did not notice because of your subjective involvement.

PROCESS RECORDING

Date **Client** **Time**

Nurse

Place

Significant Environmental Factors

Long-term Goals

Short-term Goals

Description of Client

Preconceptions

Client Behavior and Response	Nurse Behavior and Response	Interpretation and Conclusions

UNIT 4

Beginning the Data Base: Client Profile, Family, Home, and Community Assessment

OBJECTIVES

When you have completed this unit you should be able to:

1. Describe the following parts of a problem-oriented health record:
   a. client profile
   b. problem list
   c. initial plans
   d. progress notes
2. Collect data, by interviewing, for a client profile, and for family, home, and community assessments.
3. Draw a client's family structure.

PROBLEM-ORIENTED HEALTH RECORDS

In Unit 1 you learned that client charts or medical records could be organized according to the problem-oriented method. Now you are about to begin using this system to organize the data of your nursing assessments. To help you put the assessments into perspective, you should know how a complete problem-oriented health record is organized. The parts of a problem-oriented health record are (1) the data base, (2) a problem list, (3) the initial plans, and (4) progress notes. Each of these is explained briefly below.

1. Data Base

Just as the first step in problem solving is always collecting information, the first step in creating a POHR is establishing a data base. The exact contents of the data base depend on the purposes for which it will be used (for example, teaching and research institutions usually require a more detailed data base), the level of skill and professional education of the practitioners writing the data base, the time available to collect data, and other factors. Both subjective and objective data are collected for the data base. Usually the data base is composed of (1) background information on the client, his family, and his community, (2) the client's history of past and present health problems and health maintenance activities, (3) the findings of the physical and mental examination, and (4) the results of laboratory tests.

2. Problem List

The problem list is developed as a result of the next step in problem solving—interpretation of the data base. Problems are identified as described in Unit 2 and listed on a special page, placed at the front of the POHR. As problems are identified, they are given a name, numbered sequentially, dated, and written onto the problem list. The problem list becomes the first page or pages of the client's health record and serves as a kind of table of contents for the rest of the chart. The problem-list page also has a column for noting when and/or how a problem is resolved or becomes inactive for one reason or another.

3. Initial Plans

Only after the preceding steps have been completed is the health professional ready to proceed to the next step—writing plans for working on the identified problems. Each practitioner utilizes his or her knowledge of health and illness, and interpersonal and technical skills to formulate plans. All health professionals follow the same format in writing up their plans. This makes it easier to find out what each practitioner working with a client plans to contribute to the client's total care. Initial plans are discussed more completely in Unit 7.

4. Progress Notes

To complete the problem-solving process and provide feedback for improving the care of the client, all plans are evaluated by collecting and analyzing new data. The record of this process is contained in the section called *progress notes.* Progress notes describe what happens after the initial plans are implemented. They describe changes in the client's condition, evaluate whether or not the initial plans are producing the planned effects, and state whether the plans are to be continued or new ones formulated.

Like initial plans, progress notes are dated and labeled with the problem name and number to which they are addressed. This means it is possible to follow a particular problem all the way through a client's chart, from the first page (problem list), through the initial plans, through however many progress notes are added as the plans succeed or fail. It would be much more difficult to find all the information pertaining to one problem in a traditionally organized chart, since you would have to look through all the physician's notes, all the nurses' notes, and so on.

Narrative progress notes follow the format of Subjective (data), Objective (data), Assessment (of the data), and Plans. This will be explained in Unit 8. Another way of noting new data, interpretations, and plans is through the use of flow sheets. These specially designed charts are explained in Unit 5.

As you proceed through the assessment practice exercises in this workbook, you will be developing parts of a POHR for your client or clients. This text contains a fairly complete data-base outline for nursing assessment. After collecting the data, you should interpret your findings, identify any problems, list the problems on a problem list, write initial plans, and—whenever it is possible to evaluate the outcome of your interventions—write progress notes.

THE CLIENT PROFILE, FAMILY, HOME, AND COMMUNITY ASSESSMENT

For your first assessment, you will be interviewing to obtain information that will tell you what norms to apply when interpreting all the additional data throughout the remainder of the data base. These very basic data are called the *client profile* because they help you know the client better as an individual. A complete client profile will give you a great deal of information about your client and his everyday life as seen from his point of view. This will be valuable later when you try to interpret how health problems affect your client and his lifestyle.

Immediately following the client profile is a *family, home,* and *community assessment.* You need this information right away as you begin your assessments, since these, too, are influences which will have to be taken into account throughout the remainder of the problem-solving process. Although the data for the family, home, and community assessments are usually collected by interviewing the client, more objective (and sometimes more complete and accurate) data can be obtained if you are able to make some direct observations. Visiting the client in his home, for example, would provide you with an opportunity to observe behavior of family members and to see the community for yourself. What happens if your own assessment differs from what your client told you during the interview? The most helpful way of using this finding would be to record what the client told you as subjective data; then follow this with your own description, being as objective and nonjudgmental as you can. Be sure to clearly label which is the client's description and which is your own.

Sometimes in the course of interviewing a client, it becomes clear that he is—for whatever reason—providing false or misleading information. For this reason, a notation is made in the beginning of the data base as to who is the source of the information and whether or not the person seems reliable as a health historian. Any information obtained from a previously compiled health record should be identified as such.

ASSESSMENT PRACTICE

You are now ready to begin your data base by writing a client profile, and a family and community assessment. You will be most successful if you utilize interviewing techniques that create a climate in which your client can feel free to give you the information you need. When asking open-ended questions such as "Tell me how you spend an average day," or "Describe a typical day from when you wake up in the morning till you go to bed in the evening," it is helpful to be prepared to ask more specific questions if the client tends to become overly involved in one aspect of his reply or only talks about part of the day's activities. If the client has difficulty understanding what you mean by a "typical" or "average" day or is vague in his response, ask him to describe the day previous to the interview. Similarly, you may need to structure responses to questions such as "Tell me about your social life" by asking additional questions like "Tell me about your friends" or "What do you like to do for fun?" Keeping in mind the purpose behind this data collection—to understand the social and environmental factors that influence the client's health—should help you to plan how to phrase questions and to know how much detail is desirable in the client's responses. Remember, too, that it is not necessary to collect the data in exactly the same order in which you will record it. If you follow the data collection outline too rigidly, you may miss important information that the client might volunteer if allowed some freedom of expression. The readings suggested in the bibliography that follows give more information on the purposes of the assessment, and the readings in Unit 3 can help you with interviewing skills.

SELECTED BIBLIOGRAPHY

The Problem-Oriented Record

Becknell, Eileen Pearlman, and Dorothy M. Smith: *System of Nursing Practice,* F.A. Davis, Philadelphia, 1975, pp. 15-17.

Berni, Rosemarian: "The Problem-Oriented Record," in Ann Marriner, *The Nursing Process,* C.V. Mosby, St. Louis, 1975, pp. 43-55.

Mitchell, Pamela Holsclaw: *Concepts Basic to Nursing,* McGraw-Hill, New York, 1977, pp. 160–171.

Van Meeter, Margie J.: "Problem-Oriented Documentation of Nursing Practice," in Josephine M. Sana and Richard D. Judge (eds.), *Physical Appraisal Methods in Nursing Practice,* Little, Brown, Boston, 1975, pp. 25-38.

Weed, Lawrence: "Medical Records That Guide and Teach," *New England Journal of Medicine,* **278**:593-600, March 14, 1968.

Woody, Mary, and Mary Mallison: "The Problem-Oriented System for Patient-Centered Care," *American Journal of Nursing,* **73**:1168-1175, 1973.

Health and Family

Mitchell, Pamela Holsclaw: *Concepts Basic to Nursing,* McGraw-Hill, New York, 1977, pp. 189–203, 209–210.

Health and Environment

Mitchell, Pamela Holsclaw: *Concepts Basic to Nursing,* McGraw-Hill, New York, 1977, pp. 242–249.

DATE:

ASSESSMENT PRACTICE 6: Client Profile[1]

Try to obtain all the information by interviewing. Use health records only when necessary. Always indicate the source of information.

Source(s) and reliability of data

Client name

Age Sex Birthdate

Ethnicity and place of birth

Occupation

Religious practices

Level of education

Language spoken and ability to read and write

Health-related personal habits (use of alcohol, caffeine, cigarettes, any over-the-counter or "street" drugs, nail biting, or other habits)

Pattern of socialization and description of friends

Activity-rest pattern: how client spends an average day (be specific)

What are client's current health goals?

[1] Reprinted with permission of the Herbert H. Lehman College Department of Nursing, Data Base Collection Outline, Problem Oriented-Family Health Record, 1975.

DATE:

ASSESSMENT PRACTICE 7: Family Assessment[2]

Client's marital history

With whom does client live now?

Client's position, role in family

Reproductive data (number of pregnancies, living children, contraceptive methods if applicable, menstrual patterns, including menarche and menopause if applicable)

Availability and use of nonhousehold family members and significant others: relationships with neighbors and other community members

Anything else client views as significant about family

Economic status

Amount and sources of income

Sources of health care payment

Adequacy of economic resources to meet current needs

[2] Adapted from and used by permission of the Herbert H. Lehman College Department of Nursing, Data Base Collection Outline, Problem-Oriented Family Health Record, 1975.

DATE:

ASSESSMENT PRACTICE 8: Home and Community Assessment[3]

Living Conditions

Brief description of home by client and/or interviewer: type of dwelling; cooking/eating, bathing, and sleeping arrangements; sanitation—vermin, plumbing, garbage; safety locks, bars at windows; chipping paint and plaster; other factors related to specific health problems such as number of stairs to climb, presence of pets, lighting, ventilation, and screening.

Is environment suited to client's health needs? Describe.

[3]Reprinted with permission of the Herbert H. Lehman College Department of Nursing, Data Base Collection Outline, Problem-Oriented Family Health Record, 1975.

Community Assessment

Physical structures in community (high-rise apartments, single-family homes, farm buildings)

Population characteristics (ethnic, age, social class)

Availability and use of community facilities

Shopping

Recreation

Religious

Social and cultural

Transportation available to above and to health and social service agencies

DATE:

ASSESSMENT PRACTICE 9: Family Structure: Genetic History

Draw the client's family tree, including that person's generation, parents and grandparents, and children, if any. Under each person's first name, write his or her age or date of death, and any significant health problems known. These would include allergies, alcoholism, obesity, mental illness, arthritis, high blood pressure, heart disease, for example. See the example and code below.

Code

0 = female

□ = male

0—□ = mating

a & w = alive, well

d = died

Example

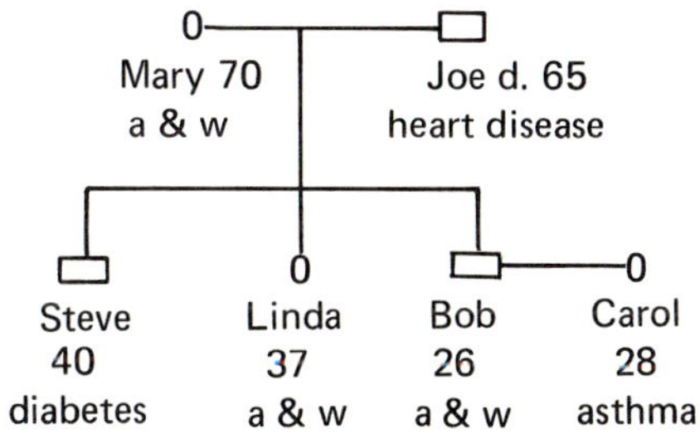

UNIT 5

Health History

OBJECTIVES

When you have completed this unit, you should be able to:

1. Explain the components of a health history:
   a. present health history
   b. past health history
   c. review of systems
2. List the data to be collected about past and present problems (signs or symptoms) reported by the client.
3. Utilize a flow sheet to record health maintenance data.

HEALTH HISTORY

The subjective data in a complete data base consist of the *health history,* which has several components. (1) The *present health history* is a summary of information about the "chief complaint"—the present problem for which the client is seeking health care services. The client profile and family structure, which were introduced in Unit 4, are also part of the present health history. (2) The *past health history* provides the practitioner with information about the client's previous illnesses and injuries and his ways of coping with these. (3) The *review of systems,* often abbreviated to ROS, is a systematic review of possible problems related to all the major organ systems of the body and including mental functioning. The purpose of this comprehensive, systematic approach is to minimize the chance of overlooking significant but previously unnoticed signs or symptoms.

HISTORY OF PRESENT PROBLEM: CHIEF COMPLAINT

Practitioners usually begin taking the health history by questioning the client about his general state of health and the signs or symptoms that are his main concern. The *chief complaint* is the main reason why the client is seeking help at this time; it should be stated concisely and in the client's own words, if possible. (Note that the client's chief complaint may or may not correspond to the data considered most important by the health care practitioner.) If the client's reason for seeking health care is a health maintenance activity such as an annual checkup rather than a specific health problem, this is noted in the client's health record in place of the chief complaint.

After questioning the client about the chief complaint and assessing his general appearance, the practitioner must set priorities for proceeding with the remaining parts of the health history. In an emergency room, with a client in acute distress, the practitioner would probably combine history taking with examination, and defer most of the client profile and family and community assessments until a later time. In other situations, such as a long-term care facility or well-child clinic, the practitioner often begins the health history with the client profile, which serves as a basis for assessing health maintenance needs and goals.

Interviewing methods such as the use of general, open-ended questions are usually effective in helping the client describe his major concerns. Most clients can describe fairly accurately what they see as happening to them if they feel accepted and at ease in the interview. One method of establishing this comfortable climate is to really listen to the client. Privacy, if at all possible, is important both for confidentiality and to allow you and the client to concentrate on what is being said.

The *present problem* is an elaboration by the client of his chief complaint. Some basic information should be obtained about each sign or symptom reported by the client, including:

1. *Onset:* when, where, and how the problem began
2. *Course:* the development of the sign or symptom over time
3. *Duration:* length of time the problem was experienced
4. *Character:* what it looks like, feels like, to have the problem
5. *Aggravating, relieving, and associated factors:* anything else the client sees as relating to the problem
6. *Treatment and results of treatment:* what treatment was used or prescribed and how effective (This includes over-the-counter drugs and "home" remedies.)

The following example consists of part of a history-taking interview, with the nurse obtaining data about the present problem using the guidelines given above.

Client: I've been having really bad headaches lately.
Nurse: When did the headaches start?
Client: I think around six months ago.
Nurse: What are the headaches like?
Client: They're mostly around my forehead, and they come every two to three days, usually in the evening. They're very sharp and last a couple of hours.
Nurse: Do you feel any different when you have the headaches, besides feeling the pain?
Client: Most of the time I feel sick to my stomach, but that goes away when the pain goes away.
Nurse: Does anything help to relieve the pain?
Client: I take two aspirin but that doesn't really help. If I take a stiff drink or go out for a walk, sometimes that helps. I never used to drink, but since I got this job I need something to relax me.
Nurse: Does anything special or different happen before you have the headaches—like getting overtired?
Client: No.... Well, I changed jobs about eight months ago. I never had these headaches before that. It seems like a lot of things have been happening since then. I've put on weight, also. I like to keep my weight down because I know that's better for my health.

In listening carefully to the client as he describes his signs and symptoms, past health problems, and how he has coped with them, you may also hear him describing his strengths. Often, in initial interviews, health professionals may concentrate more on identifying problems and illnesses and may not "hear" the client as he also describes some of his strengths. Both strengths and problems are considered when planning health care with clients. An example of a strength in the interview above would be the client's interest in keeping his weight down in order to maintain his health.

SELECTED BIBLIOGRAPHY

Assessment Skills

Becknell, Eileen Pearlman, and Dorothy M. Smith: *System of Nursing Practice,* F.A. Davis, Philadelphia, 1975, pp. 35-59.

Marsden, Alice, and Josephine M. Sana: "Nurse-Patient Communication and Relationship in the Physical Appraisal Process," in Josephine M. Sana and Richard D. Judge (eds.), *Physical Appraisal in Nursing Practice,* Little, Brown, Boston, 1975, pp. 65-78.

Mitchell, Pamela Holsclaw: *Concepts Basic to Nursing,* McGraw-Hill, New York, 1977, pp. 85–97.

Neelon, Francis A., and George J. Ellis: *A Syllabus of Problem-Oriented Patient Care,* Little, Brown, Boston, 1974, pp. 66-71.

Prior, John A., and Jack S. Silberstein: *Physical Diagnosis,* C. V. Mosby, St. Louis, 1973, pp. 2-46.

Sherman, Jacques L., and Sylvia Kleiman Fields: *Guide to Patient Evaluation,* Medical Examination Publishing, Flushing, N.Y., 1974, pp. 19-34.

"Patient Assessment: Taking a Patient's History," Programmed Instruction, *American Journal of Nursing,* **74**:293-324, 1974.

DATE:

ASSESSMENT PRACTICE 10: Data Collection for a Present Problem

Assume a client, when asked about his general health and about any specific concerns, states: "Nothing I eat agrees with me."

Write five questions you could ask for an assessment of this problem as part of the history of present health problems. Use the guidelines presented in this unit.

DATE:

ASSESSMENT PRACTICE 11: Chief Complaint and History of Present Problem

By interviewing and consultation, try to learn about your client's present problem(s). Record the data as concisely as you can while maintaining accuracy.

Problem stated in client's own words

Onset

Course

Duration

Character

Aggravating, relieving, associated factors

Treatment and results of treatment

DATE:

ASSESSMENT PRACTICE 12: Past Health History

PAST HEALTH HISTORY

After gathering information about the client's present history, and before beginning a specific review of his health status, it is helpful to obtain a general picture of his *past health history.* This helps you to see how the client's present problem fits into his overall health pattern and if past problems may be contributing to current difficulties. The past health history includes a review of all past illnesses, accidents, hospitalizations and/or emergency room visits, and allergies.

By interviewing and consultation, try to learn about your client's past health history. Record the data as concisely as possible.

Past illnesses (childhood and adulthood)

Accidents

Hospitalizations

Emergency room visits

Travel (outside the country or to areas of known health risk)

Blood transfusions

Allergies

HEALTH PATTERNS ASSESSMENT OR REVIEW OF SYSTEMS

This part of the health history involves a systematic review of physical and mental functioning. It is a comprehensive review of all current and past problems related to each body system or pattern. It is important that this review be done thoroughly to be sure that no significant data have been overlooked by the client or practitioner. In Units 6, and 9-13, we demonstrate how to conduct a systematic review of possible problems through the use of pattern assessments. A cephalocaudal approach is a helpful way to proceed with this review. Some practitioners collect information about all the body parts and organ systems before beginning the physical examination; others prefer to ask questions as they proceed with the examination. As you gain experience, you will develop your own system for this data collection. Situational factors such as the client's ability to cooperate and the amount of time available will also influence the actual data collection procedure.

HEALTH MAINTENANCE DATA

Health maintenance involves your working together with the client to help him stay healthy. Health maintenance includes teaching, preventive care, and regular assessment to detect health status changes in their early stages. Data to be collected for the health maintenance history include the client's immunizations, dental care, breast self-exam and pap smear for women, rectal exam for men, complete physical examination, vision testing, hearing testing, chest x ray and/or tuberculin test, testing for venereal disease, and contraceptive information and supplies, if applicable. The practitioner also considers information gathered elsewhere in the data base, such as smoking habits, occupation, and familial illnesses, from the client profile and family structure. It is convenient to record some of the above information on a flow sheet rather than in narrative form.

FLOW SHEETS

Flow sheets (or *flow charts*) are specially designed charts that record pertinent health status data at given intervals of time. This method of recording is more concise, faster, and often much more useful than narrative notes. Consider the differences between the two methods of recording health status data below:

Example: **Narrative Notes**

8/25/73 10 A.M. TPR = 37.6°-84-18, BP = 108/70.
Had 1 cup tea, 1 cup cream of wheat at 8 A.M. No incision pain.
8/25/73 2 P.M. Resting quietly. C/o pain in incision, meperidine (Demerol) 25 mg given IM at 1:45 P.M. Ate full liquid lunch (1 cup mushroom soup, 1/2 cup jello, 1/2 cup ice cream, 1 cup tea).
TPR = 38°-92-18, BP = 110/70
8/25/73 4 P.M. No complaints of pain. Ambulating. Pulse = 80, resp = 18.

FIGURE 5-1. EXAMPLE: FLOW SHEET

Date	Time	Subjective	TPR	BP	Intake	Comments
8/25/73	10 A.M.	No incision pain	37.6°-84-18	108/70	480 ml	
	2 P.M.	Incision pain	38°-92-18	114/72	800 ml	Meperidine 25 mg IM@1:45 P.M.
	4 P.M.	No pain	80-18	110/70		Ambulated to chair in room

It is apparent that the flow sheet allows easier comparison of changes in health status over time. Since the flow sheet lists the health status parameters to be recorded at the time intervals, it also helps prevent loss of data because a busy practitioner forgot to mention a finding in an unstructured narrative note. The medication record and graphic sheet in the sample data in Unit 1 are examples of flow sheets in common use in both traditional and problem-oriented charts.

What kinds of data can be recorded on a flow sheet? Almost any information that can be stated or summarized briefly and that changes or may change over time. Many practitioners are designing flow sheets to fit the special needs of their clients, to record information such as coronary care data, diabetic care, recovery room care. The example below is a flow sheet designed to record health maintenance data at monthly intervals. As you see, it's not necessary that all parameters be measured at each interval, but each column in the chart represents the same amount of time—one month.

FIGURE 5-2. EXAMPLE: HEALTH MAINTENANCE FLOW SHEET

Client: Robert Lafayette Age: 39

Date	6/74	7/74	8/74	9/74
Complete physical exam	done			
Blood pressure check	150/90	140/90		136/86
VDRL	nonreactive			
Tuberculin test	neg			
Dental visit			8/74 OK	
Vision testing	o.d. 20/20 o.s. 20/30			
Hearing testing	not done			
Fasting blood sugar	250			182
Weight	86.8 kg			82.7 kg

Another example of how a flow sheet may be used is shown below. This flow sheet was designed to record data of home visits made by a nurse practitioner. Flow sheets may also be utilized for progress notes (see Unit 8).

FIGURE 5-3. FLOW SHEET: RECORD OF HOME VISITS

Client: Mrs. D. Carr, Age: 45 5/75 Problem #1: Blood Sugar—220 mg

Date	Urine		FBS	Weight	Comments
	Sugar	Acetone			
6/10/75	2+	0	-	79.5 kg	Client adhering to prescribed diabetic diet
6/17/75	0	0	95	78.6 kg	FBS decreased Continues to adhere to diet
6/24/75	4+	trace	-	78.6 kg	Client discouraged about diet. Ate chocolate candy last night. See progress note of 6/24/75 for nursing plan.
7/1/75	1+	0	-	77.3 kg	Client pleased with ability to return to diet and stay with it.
7/7/75	0	0	-	77.3 kg	Client feels well. Taught to test urine for sugar and acetone.
7/14/75	0	0	-	76.8 kg	Client adhering to diet. Tests own urine. Schedule visits q. 2 weeks.

DATE:

ASSESSMENT PRACTICE 13: Use of Flow Sheet with Sample Data

The following portion of the interview includes some of the kinds of past health history and health maintenance data described on the preceding pages. Read the interview, then record the information on the flow sheet which follows. The client being interviewed is Linda Leone, age 18.

July 7, 1975

Nurse: I'd like to ask you a few questions about your past health history. Have you had any childhood illnesses like measles, mumps, or chicken pox?

Client: Yeah, I had measles when I was five. I never had polio—we got sugar cubes in the first grade that had vaccine on them so we wouldn't get polio.

Nurse: Do you remember if you had the regular measles or the German measles?

Client: It was the regular measles.

Nurse: Besides the polio vaccine, have you ever had any other immunizations?

Client: I stepped on a nail three months ago and I went to the emergency room. They gave me a tetanus shot there. I was all right. I had a smallpox vaccination last year when I went to India.

Nurse: When was the last time you had a health checkup?

Client: Two years ago I saw a doctor in the clinic. He checked me out. I had a women's exam and a chest x ray. He told me that I was anemic and that I should eat more meat and take iron pills. I don't eat meat because I'm a vegetarian, but I did take the iron pills.

Nurse: Have you been back for a further checkup on the anemia?

Client: No, I feel all right.

Nurse: So you were anemic two years ago. Did you find out if any of the other tests you had showed anything unusual?

Client: They sent me a card that said that the x ray was okay and the pap smear was okay and I didn't have any VD.

Nurse: Do you examine your breasts for lumps?

Client: No, should I?

Nurse: Yes, that's important for staying healthy. I'll show you how when you have your examination.

Client: Okay.

Nurse: When was the last time your vision was checked?

Client: Two years ago when I came to the clinic.

Nurse: How about hearing testing?

Client: I never had any.

Nurse: When was the last time you saw a dentist?

Client: When I was a kid—maybe when I was ten. Is there a dentist in this clinic?

Now record the health maintenance data from this interview on the flow sheet on the next page. Some of the data has already been entered for you.

HEALTH MAINTENANCE FLOW SHEET

Dates:	Childhood	1973	1974	1975	Normal Values
Immunizations					
DPT, TOPV, mumps, rubella, influenza, smallpox, etc. — Polio	1st grade				
Tuberculin test					
Chest x ray					
Complete physical examination					
Blood pressure					
EKG					
Dental					
Vision					
Hearing					
Pap smear					
Urinalysis					
WBC with diff					
Hgb		"anemic"			
Hct					
FBS					
Na+					
K+					
Cl^-					
CO_2					
Serology		neg			
Sickle cell trait					

Source: Reprinted with permission of the Herbert H. Lehman College Department of Nursing, Data Base Collection Outline, Problem-Oriented Family Health Record, 1975.

DATE:

ASSESSMENT PRACTICE 14: Use of Flow Sheet

Utilize interviewing and consultation methods to obtain health maintenance data for your client.

HEALTH MAINTENANCE FLOW SHEET

Dates:					Normal Values
Immunizations					
DPT, TOPV, mumps, rubella, influenza, smallpox, etc.					
Tuberculin test					
Chest x ray					
Complete physical examination					
Blood pressure					
EKG					
Dental					
Vision					
Hearing					
Pap smear					
Urinalysis					
WBC with diff					
Hgb					
Hct					
FBS					
Na+					
K+					
Cl^-					
CO_2					
Serology					
Sickle cell trait					

Source: Reprinted with permission of the Herbert H. Lehman College Department of Nursing, Data Base Collection Outline, Problem-Oriented Family Health Record, 1975.

UNIT 6

Beginning the Physical Examination: Assessment of Physical Structure

OBJECTIVES

When you have completed this unit, you should be able to:

1. Explain the purpose of physical examination as part of the data base.
2. Collect, by interviewing, a history of past and present problems related to physical structure.
3. Collect, by inspection, palpation, and consultation, objective data for a health assessment of a client's physical structure. Objective data includes:
   a. physical examination data
   b. laboratory data
   c. chart data
4. Review the data collected and enter any problems identified on the problem list.

PHYSICAL EXAMINATION

The history that precedes the physical examination provides a summary of the client's health status in all major areas of functioning. These data not only indicate which signs or symptoms need to be investigated further by physical and/or laboratory examination, but also give a sense of what the problems mean to the client and how he has attempted to deal with them. The *physical examination* consists of a systematic examination of the body using the assessment skills of inspection, auscultation, palpation, and percussion. Examination provides objective data about the person's health status and is most useful when considered along with the history data given by the client. If you and the client have reviewed his history thoroughly, you will have definite indications of what to "zero in" on when you do the physical examination. Using the cephalocaudal, midline-to-periphery approach will help you perform a complete examination in each assessment area without having to memorize a list of what to examine.

The importance of using all your senses well to collect data was mentioned in Unit 1. It goes almost without saying that you should try to eliminate as many factors as possible that would interfere with using your senses during examination. To inspect well you must have good light, since without it you might not be able to see the discoloration of the skin caused by poor oxygenation or liver disease. A noisy environment, or one that allows many interruptions to distract you and/or the client, will also interfere with accurate observations.

You will have to ask the client to remove clothing that interferes with examination: you cannot inspect a wound or palpate skin temperature or auscultate a blood pressure through bedsheets or clothing. Privacy and your own matter-of-fact, assured manner (having gained competency in the skills practicing with peers helps), will make the necessary intimacy less uncomfortable for both of you. If you are examining a client while giving nursing care such as assisting with bathing or dressing, it may not be necessary to ask the client to undress for the specific purpose of examination. On the other hand, if you are performing an examination in a clinic, you might have to ask the client to remove clothing (except underpants or shorts) and put on a hospital-style gown.

HISTORY AND PHYSICAL EXAMINATION FOR PHYSICAL STRUCTURE

Using the guidelines presented in this unit and preceding ones, you should now be able to collect a health history and perform an examination in the assessment area of physical structure. These assessment practice exercises allow you to evaluate the client's physical outer boundaries—skin and mucous membranes, visible body structure, and appearance. When you evaluate personal hygiene, you will also learn more about the client's health maintenance practices. Before you initiate this or other history-taking interviews, you should read through the list of data to be collected and, if necessary, review the normal anatomy and physiology related to that assessment. A good understanding of what is normal and healthy is essential so that you will know what norms to apply when interpreting your data. Since you will want to ask for specific information about actual or potential problems (onset, location, influencing factors, etc.) it will be to your advantage to begin to identify unusual or abnormal findings early in the data collection process.

As part of Assessment Practice 1, you wrote an objective description of a person, using the skill of inspection to gather your data. You cannot, of course, perform a complete examination of the physical structure of a person using inspection alone, since you cannot see through the skin. Laboratory data from x-ray examinations is one means of gathering more complete data; another is to use the physical assessment skills of palpation, auscultation, and percussion. You will begin to use the skill of auscultation when you assess oxygenation. Beginning practitioners can use the skill of palpation on the head, by palpating the skull for bumps, soft spots, or other irregularities. This will also allow you to note the amount and texture of the hair. You may already have realized that assisting a client with activities of daily living such as bathing and dressing provides an excellent opportunity to use the skills of inspection and palpation for assessment of physical structure.

Begin your written description of the client's physical structure with a summary of the client's general appearance. This should indicate whether the client looks old, young, or about average for his given age, whether he is over- or under-weight, if physical development seems appropriate for the age, and any obvious physical deformities.

RECORDING YOUR FINDINGS FOR HISTORY AND PHYSICAL EXAMINATION

There are a few "rules" you should keep in mind as you write up your findings from the history and physical examination:

1. *Be concise.* Don't use extra words.
2. *Be objective.* If you are stating your own or someone else's opinion rather than what was actually observed, say so.

3. *Be accurate.* If you are not sure of a finding, recheck it if at all possible, or consider that portion of the assessment incomplete until you have rechecked. Write, "not observed" or, "not done."
4. *Be complete.* In the complete data base, there should be some kind of notation for each bit of information you are seeking.

Here are some samples for reporting data about allergies:

1. Client reports allergies to penicillin and tomatoes.
2. Client reports no allergies known.
3. Unable to determine if client has allergies.

ASSESSMENT PRACTICE

If you have looked ahead in this book or used some of the suggested readings, you may have noticed that the assessments are not always organized strictly "system by system," but fall instead into broader assessment areas, or health patterns, such as physical structure, mobility/comfort/rest, oxygenation, nutrition/elimination, and mental, emotional, and sensory status. This approach will help you learn the skills while still considering the whole person and is more in line with the major goal of nursing assessment—to discover problems of response to illness, rather than to make differential diagnoses of specific diseases.

SELECTED BIBLIOGRAPHY

Assessment Skills

Crane, Joyce: "Physical Appraisal: An Aspect of the Nursing Assessment," in Josephine M. Sana and Richard D. Judge (eds.), *Physical Appraisal Methods in Nursing Practice,* Little, Brown, Boston, 1975, pp. 11-24.

Fuerst, Ellnor V., LuVerne Wolff, and Marlene H. Weitzel: *Fundamentals of Nursing,* 5th ed., J. B. Lippincott, Philadelphia, 1974, pp. 205-214.

Skin and Physical Structure Assessment

Bates, Barbara: *A Guide to Physical Examination,* J. B. Lippincott, Philadelphia, 1974, pp. 8-16, 17-29, 73-80, 145-147, 154-155, 158-160, 179-180, 188-189.

Brown, Marie Scott, and Mary Alexander: "Physical Examination, Part 3, Examining the Skin," *Nursing '73,* **3**:39-43, September 1973.

Derbes, Vincent J.: "Skin Rashes: Recognition and Management," *Nursing '73,* **3**:44-49, March 1973.

Fuerst, Elinor V., LuVerne Wolff, and Marlene H. Weitzel: *Fundamentals of Nursing,* J. B. Lippincott, Philadelphia, 1974, pp. 243-267.

Mitchell, Pamela Holsclaw: *Concepts Basic to Nursing,* McGraw-Hill, 1977, pp. 493–521.

Roach, Lora B.: "Assessing Skin Changes—the Subtle and the Obvious," *Nursing '74,* **4**:64-69, March 1974.

Roberts, Sharon L.: "Skin Assessment for Color and Temperature," *American Journal of Nursing,* **75**:610-613, 1975.

Sherman, Jacques L., and Sylvia Kleiman Fields: *Guide to Patient Evaluation,* Medical Examination Publishing, Flushing, N.Y., 1974, pp. 50-62.

DATE:

ASSESSMENT PRACTICE 15: Health History for Physical Structure

Use interviewing to obtain this data. What the client tells you is subjective data, which will guide the next stage of your examination.

History (subjective data)

1. Does the client now have or has he ever had in the past:
   - **a.** skin changes (rashes, lesions, infections, any other changes)
   - **b.** nail changes (breaking, brittle, color change)
   - **c.** hair changes
   - **d.** bone fracture
   - **e.** swelling or other change in body part
   - **f.** loss or deformity of body part
2. Does client use any prostheses (dentures, artificial limb) or supportive devices such as cane, crutches, built-up shoe?
3. Client's usual hygiene habits (bathing, brushing teeth, hair care, nail care).
4. Client's knowledge of hygiene needs (your evaluation based on information in (3) above).
5. Is the client using any medications for his skin (soaps, ointments), or any medications in relation to any problems he has stated? Include summary of client's understanding of medications.

DATE:

ASSESSMENT PRACTICE 16: Examination of Physical Structure

Use the skills of inspection and palpation to assess physical structure. The data you obtain by looking and touching is objective data. Consultation may also be helpful, for example, to obtain information from the chart.

Physical Examination (objective data)

1. *Statement of general appearance.*
   Briefly describe client by shape/build, size/proportions, symmetry of body parts, apparent age, and/or a few other phrases which would distinguish him from others in a waiting room.

2. *Skin and hair.*
   You can examine skin and hair as you proceed in cephalocaudal manner to assess body structures. For example, as you examine the head, you would assess the skin of the face and scalp, and note hair condition and distribution. What to check for in skin assessment: color, lesions, scars, birthmarks, cleanliness, texture, turgor, temperature, wetness-dryness, intactness. Remember to include a skin assessment in each area of the physical structure assessment.

3. *Head*
   a. shape/proportion

   b. irregularities or asymmetry of face and skull

   c. hair color, distribution, texture

   d. skin

4. *Eyes*

	Right	*Left*
a. eyebrows present		
b. eyelids (drooping, lashes present)		
c. conjunctiva (color)		
d. sclerae (color)		
e. iris (color)		
f. pupils (color, shape, equality)		

5. *Ears*
   a. symmetry

   b. presence of wax, discharge

6. *Nose*
   a. shape, symmetry on face

   b. discharge

7. *Mouth*
   a. symmetry

   b. color of lips, condition

   c. tongue (color, hydration)

   d. teeth (condition, hygiene)

   e. gums (color, condition)

   f. buccal mucosa (hydration, color)

8. *Neck*
   a. symmetry

   b. skin

9. *Chest*
   a. deformities of thorax (barrel-shaped chest, "pigeon" breast)

   b. skin

10. *Breasts*
    a. development (relative to age)

    b. symmetry, shape

    c. nipple discharge

    d. skin

11. *Back*
    a. contour (deformities such as kyphosis, scoliosis)

    b. skin

12. *Abdomen*
    a. contour (protuberant, flat)

    b. scars

    c. skin

13. *Genitalia, male*

Note developmental status, skin and hair, any swelling or discharge of:

a. penis

b. urethra

c. scrotum

d. rectum

14. *Genitalia, female*

Note developmental status, skin and hair, any swelling or discharge of:

a. labia majora and minora

b. urethra

c. vaginal opening

d. rectum

15. *Extremities*

	Right	*Left*
arms and hands		
a. symmetry		
b. joint swelling		
c. skin		
d. nails (color, shape, mobility)		
legs and feet		
a. symmetry		
b. varicosities		
c. joint swelling		
d. skin		
e. nails		

Laboratory Data

Any x-ray reports indicating normal or abnormal structure (such as enlarged heart, healed fracture)

Medications Related to Physical Structure

Check chart, Kardex, physician's order sheet to validate client's drug, dose, route of administration, when given.[1]

[1] Beginning students may want to include expected effects of the drug.

DATE:

ASSESSMENT PRACTICE 17: Problem List

INTERPRETING YOUR DATA AND IDENTIFYING PROBLEMS

Establishing the defined data base is the first step in problem solving. When you have collected the data, you are ready to compare your findings with the appropriate norms and make judgments about actual or potential problems. You may want to review the section explaining this part of the problem-solving process in Unit 2. Inspect your own data base and determine which of your data represent normal findings for the client and which indicate actual or potential health problems. List any problems identified by you or the client from the data you have collected up to now on the problem list that follows. If the data base indicates normal, healthy findings, consider various health maintenance needs in the area assessed. Also list any health maintenance "problems" on the problem list. Remember that the problem list becomes page one of the POHR even though it is not the first step in problem solving.

PROBLEM LIST

Date Identified	Date of Onset	Problem Number	Problem Title	Date Inactive/ Resolved

UNIT 7

Initial Plans for Nursing Intervention

OBJECTIVES

When you have completed this unit, you should be able to:

1. Explain in your own words the rationale for recording nursing plans in writing.
2. Explain the development of initial plans for intervention as the third step of the problem-solving process.
3. Write initial plans for problems identified including:
   a. subjective data about problems
   b. objective data about problems
   c. assessment of the problem
   d. diagnostic plans
   e. therapeutic plans
   f. client teaching plans
   g. referral plans

INITIAL PLANS AND NURSING INTERVENTIONS

When you and the client have clearly defined a problem, you can begin to use your knowledge of facts and theories and your own creativity to propose nursing interventions designed to solve the problem. This step of the problem-solving process is written into the POHR together with the data base and problem list. In the problem-oriented record-keeping system, the *initial plan* format is designed to encourage the practitioner to base the plan on available data and communicate it clearly to professional colleagues as well as to clients and their families. The written record of planning for intervention also makes it possible to evaluate whether specific plans have been carried out as proposed and to feed back information about their effectiveness.

It is not the purpose of this workbook to suggest plans that might be effective for specific problems. Nursing books, articles in nursing and other professional journals, and audio-visual aids are available to meet this need. It is impossible to overemphasize the usefulness of the skill of consultation, which helps you discover how other nurses or other health professionals have tried to resolve a problem. As you become more knowledgeable and experienced yourself, you will still use this skill when less experienced colleagues consult with you!

HOW TO WRITE AN INITIAL PLAN

As the name indicates, an initial plan is the first plan written for each problem on the list. There is only one initial plan; once this plan has been entered into the record, all subsequent data, diagnoses, and plans related to a particular problem are recorded as progress notes, which will be explained in the next unit. Working through the following steps will help you formulate your initial plans.

1. Label the plan with the date, time, number, and name of the problem, and the designation "initial plan."

2. Consider your subjective data pertaining to the problem. All symptoms reported by the client are part of the subjective data. Write a brief summary of these subjective data (S.). Examples of such summaries are: (a) "Reports chest pain and shortness of breath after climbing stairs," or (b) a direct quote such as "I have nightmares and cannot sleep well without sleeping pills."

3. Consider the objective data pertaining to the problem. What data have you obtained from your own observations, examination of the client, consultation with other professionals, and the client's health records, laboratory data, physician's orders? Write a summary of these objective data (O.). Examples of summaries of objective data are: (a) "Apical rate 82/min and regular. No murmur." or (b) "Wearing same clothing, soiled and wrinkled, as on last visit. Speaks in short phrases or nods or shakes head. Clutching rosary in right hand."

4. The next step of the initial plan, the assessment step (A.), is a most important one, for it is here that you state your own thoughts about the problem. The assessment is a summary of your interpretation of the subjective and objective data. In it, you may include one or more of the following: (1) a probable explanation for why the problem exists and what other potential problems might result from it, (2) significant positive and negative factors that may influence solving the problem, (examples: age, economic factors, client's desire to remain independent), (3) the significance of this problem to the client's health status, and (4) an explanation of the rationale for the proposed intervention and what you expect to happen as a result. At this point in the problem-solving process, you may need to refer to literature in nursing and related fields for theory and research findings to supplement your own experience and knowledge.

The assessment part of the plan indicates your understanding of the data at the time it is written, and its complexity will depend on how well you understand the problem. Sometimes the assessment may simply consist of a restatement of the problem, e.g., "weight loss, cause undetermined." Such an assessment would logically lead to a plan of collecting additional data. An example of an assessment that sets priorities for problem solving might be "persistent high fever is life-threatening." This would logically lead to plans to bring the body temperature down as soon as possible. Both of these assessment statements provide the rationale for nursing intervention. In summary then, the assessment is the part of the plan that indicates how you, the practitioner, are viewing the problem, and presents your rationale for the initiation of nursing intervention. The assessment is always recorded as part of the written initial plan.

5. The plan (P.), the proposed intervention/management of the problem, usually has three parts, (1) diagnostic, (2) therapeutic, and (3) client teaching. At times, a fourth part may be indicated, that of referral. Initial plans written by nurses are in actuality "nursing orders," that is, statements of how to manage or intervene in the client's problem, specifying exactly what is to be done, by whom, where, and when.

While any member of the health team may read them, nursing plans are directed toward nursing care. The different parts of the initial plan are listed below.

1. *Diagnostic.* In many cases, you will need to collect additional data to evaluate the possibilities of different causes of the problem stated in the assessment. You may also need to talk further with the client about how he or she views the problem. Diagnostic plans state specifically what you plan to do to gather more information. Some examples of diagnostic plans are: (a) Check results of Hgb and Hct (blood drawn this A.M.). (b) Confer with physical therapist as to what ROM exercises client may continue to do on unit. (c) Discuss with client this afternoon what health goals he has for ADL.
2. *Therapeutic.* Here you state specifically what you and the client will try to do in one or more of the following areas: (1) alleviate the problem and/or its symptoms and side effects, (2) prevent further complications, (3) help the client maintain, restore, or learn new patterns of coping with the problem. Therapeutic plans state nursing interventions in specific areas that relate to and affect the problem (examples: ADL, nutrition, pharmacology, environmental factors, acute and chronic care regimens, family involvement, and mental and emotional status). The client's strengths should be considered and utilized in the formulation of the plan. Remember that the nursing order in the plan must be clearly stated. Nonspecific terms such as "provide emotional support" need to be clarified. If an elderly client talks consistently of "being of no use anymore," your nursing plan might specify "listen to client's reminiscences of her past school teacher days and family life." Similarly a nursing plan to "prevent decubiti" needs to be more specifically written as "Turn and position client q. 2 h (even). See turning chart at bedside." Other examples of therapeutic plans might be: (a) apply lotion to reddened area under left breast q.d. after bath 10 A.M., (b) both side rails up on bed h.s., and (c) give 8 oz orange or grapefruit juice at 9 P.M. q.d.
3. *Teaching.* This part of the plan involves what you will teach the client and family about the problem and treatment. This could involve information and teaching about what the client wants and needs to know about the problem (example: diabetes, heart disease, depression), and what the family needs to know to help the client manage once he or she leaves the health care facility. Teaching plans may include diet, medications, activity, diagnostic tests, treatments, and return visits to the health care practitioner and/or health care facility. It is important to write in your plan exactly what you have told, or plan to tell, the client and family. This is one way of assuring that the client and family get the necessary information and letting all other members of the health team know what has been taught. In this way, instructions can be reinforced, and conflicting and duplicating information avoided. Some examples of teaching plans are: (a) Client taught how to transfer from wheelchair to bed. Client returned demonstration well. I will repeat teaching tomorrow afternoon when client's wife visits and demonstrate to her how she may assist client in transfer if necessary. (b) Mr. Forr to be discharged in three days. Discussed with him beginning symptoms of depression—loss of appetite, early morning awakening, withdrawal behavior, lack of interest in job, and suggested he contact Dr. Rogers or myself in walk-in clinic should these symptoms occur before scheduled return visit to clinic on 10/13/75. (c) Reviewed basic four groups of food with client in planning daily menus for self and family.

4. *Referral.* If needed, you might also include a referral plan describing the action you take to assure follow-up of the problem. This referral could be, for example, an oral report to the head nurse or a written referral for medical consultation. If the client is being discharged from a health care facility, a referral may be written to nursing personnel in community agencies such as the Visiting Nurse Service or Public Health Department for follow-up care at home. Examples of nursing referral plans include: (a) request consultation with Ms. Goldman, nurse-clinician, re client's delusions of food being poisoned, and (b) notify Dr. Matthews immediately if diastolic BP falls below 60.

The acronym "S.O.A.P." is used to help remember steps of the plan:

S. = Subjective data — Note that these are not always written out. They usually
O. = Objective data — are in teaching schools/hospitals.
A. = Assessment
P. = Plans

The following is an example of an initial plan, with all steps written out.

Initial Plan

11/6/75 10 A.M. #3 Decreased range of motion in fingers of both hands.

S. "My fingers are stiff. I don't use them much anymore."

O. Sits in room all day watching TV, participates in no other activities. ROM evaluation: Active: Unable to fully extend fingers on both hands. Passive: Reports pain with extension to full ROM. No swelling, redness. Hands and fingers cool to touch. Has difficulty with fine movements of ADL (see chart).

A. Decreased range of motion in fingers associated with decreased activity. Further loss of joint mobility and loss of muscle strength are potential problems if activity level remains low.[1] Since fine movements of ADL are already affected, a progressive loss of self-care ability could lead not only to decreased independence but also to decreased self-esteem. Passive extension of fingers still possible, but pain is present when doing so. This could influence client's desire to perform exercises. ROM exercises indicated at this point to maintain ADL status and prevent contractures.

P. *Diagnostic:*

1. Determine whether there has been change in activity, will talk with client this afternoon re previous activities prior to entering nursing home.
2. Reexamine finger ROM after bathing hands in warm water.
3. Check and record finger ROM weekly on Tuesday.

Therapeutic:

1. Assist with ADL she is currently unable to perform—buttons, zippers, shoelaces, cutting meat.
2. Begin daily ROM (passive) exercises for fingers of both hands during bath—q.d. 10 A.M.

[1] "Through a process of fibrosis, muscle and joint mobility is decreased or lost when these structures are not used." Pamela Holsclaw Mitchell, *Concepts Basic to Nursing,* McGraw-Hill, New York, 1977, p. 301. If inactivity of fingers continues, fibrosis can lead to progressive shortening of muscle, which in turn may lead to formation of contractures.

Teaching:

1. Explained purpose of ROM exercises today—to prevent stiffness, contractures, and to maintain use of hands and fingers.
2. Plan to teach client to perform exercises herself on 11/8/75.

Referral:

1. Discuss above plan with HN to provide continuity of care.
2. Plan written in Kardex.
3. Consult with O.T. about activities possible for client with her current limited ROM.

K. Quincey R.N.

SELECTED BIBLIOGRAPHY

Planning Nursing Intervention

Becknell, Eileen Pearlman, and Dorothy M. Smith: *System of Nursing Practice,* F. A. Davis, Philadelphia, 1975, pp. 85-102.

McCloskey, Joanne Comi: "The Problem-Oriented Record vs. the Nursing Care Plan: A Proposal," *Nursing Outlook,* **23**:492-495, August 1975.

Mitchell, Pamela Holsclaw: *Concepts Basic to Nursing,* McGraw-Hill, New York, 1977, pp. 129–160.

Neelon, Francis A., and George J. Ellis: *A Syllabus of Problem-Oriented Patient Care,* Little, Brown, Boston, 1974, pp. 46-53.

Van Meeter, Margie J.: "Problem-Oriented Documentation of Nursing Care," in Josephine M. Sana and Richard D. Judge (eds.), *Physical Appraisal in Nursing Practice,* Little, Brown, Boston, 1975, pp. 25-38.

Woody, Mary, and Mary Mallison: "Using the Problem-Oriented Method for Patient-Centered Care," *American Journal of Nursing,* **70**:306-310, 1970.

DATE:

ASSESSMENT PRACTICE 18: Initial Plans

Now try writing an initial plan for a problem you have identified. If you have not yet defined any problems from the data base, try writing a plan for one of the problems you found in the sample data for the client Mary Smith in Unit 2.

Date: Time: Problem # and Name:

S.

O.

A.

P. *Diagnostic:*

Therapeutic:

Teaching:

Referral:

UNIT 8

Progress Notes and Evaluation of Plans

OBJECTIVES

When you have completed this unit you should be able to:

1. Explain the use of *progress notes* as the evaluation-feedback step of the problem-solving process.
2. Write progress notes for problems with initial plans from your own data collection and from sample data using the S.O.A.P. format.

PROGRESS NOTES

You may recall from Unit 4 that the evaluation step of the problem-solving process is represented in the health record by progress notes. In this step, both you and the client evaluate what has happened since plans were implemented.

The S.O.A.P. format is again utilized, as it was in writing the initial plans. When writing progress notes, however, the S. and O. data are always written down because this is new information not available in the data base. The subjective data (S.), as always, summarize what the client states about the problem. They provide an ongoing history from the client about the problem, covering the period between the last note and the present time. It is important to note the client's observations and feelings about what is happening even though they may not agree with your own assessment. The client may also give some suggestions at this point for a change in the plans. Having to write the S. data is, therefore, an incentive to the practitioner to make problem solving a truly collaborative process with the client.

Objective data (O.) in progress notes consist of both ongoing and any *new* observations you have made about the problem since the last note was written. This could include data from lab reports, physical examination, and consultation, possibly as follow-up from your initial diagnostic plans. You might also include in your objective data what care is being initiated with the client, if this will clarify the problem, and the client's response to it. Examples of objective data are:

1. Apical rate—70, strong, regular.
2. Chest x-ray—negative.
3. Client did not maintain any eye contact with me throughout 30-minute interview.
4. Client is attending daily group meetings on unit.

The assessment (A.) part of progress notes has a purpose similar to the one in initial plans. It is a statement of your thoughts about the problem and a summary of your interpretation of the subjective and objective data. Your assessment of the problem may be different from the one in your initial plan, since new data may influence your analysis. In addition, the assessment in a progress note includes a statement of how the plan is working out in practice and what positive and negative factors are contributing to its implementation. This would include your thoughts about the client's abilities to participate in and understand the plan of care. The subjective and objective data in the progress note should support your professional judgment about the plan's effectiveness, and your assessment should state your rationale for changing, continuing, or eliminating the current nursing plan.

The ongoing nature of the problem-solving method should be apparent as you once again write plans based on the new data and evaluate the previous intervention. Plans in progress notes are similar to those in initial plans, and may include diagnostic, therapeutic, teaching, and referral parts. The plans are your directives for continuing nursing care and must be reevaluated continually in response to the status of the problem, the client's reactions to it, and the introduction of new data.

Do not be misled by the term "progress notes". It is as important to note when a nursing care plan is *not* working as to note when it is successful. Progress notes are also to state what is currently happening with a problem. For example, if you were working with a client with an elevated blood pressure, you would want to note if the blood pressure was going up or down, or remaining stable, and what, if any, variables, such as weight, anxiety, or activity, were influencing this. You might decide to record these findings in a narrative progress note, or you might decide to design a flow sheet to record the data. As explained in Unit 5, flow sheets may be utilized as progress notes. Progress notes, then, describe the current status of a particular problem as well as evaluating progress, or lack of progress.

How often progress notes are written depends on the status of the problem, the client's responses to it, the introduction of new data, and the time necessary for a plan to effect observable change. If you give acetylsalicylic acid (aspirin) to reduce a fever, you would expect to evaluate the client's response within an hour or two. But if you were teaching a client to ambulate after a CVA (stroke), you would probably evaluate the effectiveness of your approach over a period of days.There is no set number of progress notes that should be written for any given problem. Collecting new data, reevaluating, and replanning continue until the problem is resolved. Progress notes for health maintenance and preventive measures may continue indefinitely.

Here is an example of a progress note for a plan to give acetylsalicylic acid (aspirin) to reduce fever:

6/5/75 9:30 A.M. #7 Fever

S. "I feel weak but better than before."

O. TPR @ 8 A.M. = 39° (oral), 96-18
@ 9:30 A.M. = 37.8° (oral), 84-14, client perspiring, skin cool to touch.
Intake p.o. 100 cc since midnight. Lips dry, cracked.
Acetylsalicylic acid 600 mg given p.o. 8:10 A.M.

A. Fever decreased after acetylsalicylic acid given. Possibility of dehydration developing. Client feeling weak and will need help in ADL.

P. *Diagnostic:*
1. I & O

Therapeutic:

1. Continue original plan of acetylsalicylic acid 600 ml p.o. q. 4 h prn for temp ↑ 38° C
2. Check TPR q. 1 h for next 2 h then q. 4 h and prn
3. Apply lemon and glycerin to lips q.i.d. 10-2-6-10.
4. Give fluids today—to total 2000 cc by 10 P.M. (see fluid chart at bedside). Reevaluate I & O tomorrow (8 A.M.)
5. Give client bed bath.

SELECTED BIBLIOGRAPHY

Evaluating Nursing Intervention

Becknell, Eileen Pearlman, and Dorothy M. Smith: *System of Nursing Practice,* F. A. Davis, Philadelphia, 1975, pp. 103-115.

Mitchell, Pamela Holsclaw: *Concepts Basic to Nursing,* McGraw-Hill, New York, 1977, pp. 129–160.

Van Meeter, Margie J.: "Problem-Oriented Documentation of Nursing Care," in Josephine M. Sana and Richard D. Judge (eds.), *Physical Appraisal Methods in Nursing Practice,* Little, Brown, 1975, pp. 25-38.

Woody, Mary, and Mary Mallison: "Using the Problem-Oriented Method for Patient-Centered Care," *American Journal of Nursing,* **70**:306-310, 1970.

DATE:

ASSESSMENT PRACTICE 19: Progress Notes with Sample Data

Turn to Unit 7 and consult the sample initial plan. Utilize the following new data to write a progress note on this plan (problem: decreased range of motion of fingers on both hands). Your new data one week later is as follows:

1. Before admission to nursing home 3 months ago, client was quite active in quilting club.
2. Finger range of motion increases slightly after bathing hands in warm water.
3. Client states, "Your exercises are helping my fingers but I'd rather not do that myself."
4. Client still needs assistance with ADL.
5. Knitting and sewing activities available in OT.

Date: Time: Problem # and name:

S.

O.

A.

P. *Diagnostic:*

Therapeutic:

Teaching:

Referral:

Now compare your progress note with the following example. Your note will not be identical but should contain a summary of how the client now views the problem (S.), a summary of any new data and/or observations you have obtained (O.), an assessment of how the plan is working as well as the interpretation of the subjective and objective data (A.), and your plans for how you will continue to work with the problem (P.).

Progress Note

11/13/75 11 A.M. #3 Decreased range of motion in fingers of both hands

S. "Your exercises are helping my fingers but I'd rather not do them myself."

O. Active finger range of motion increases slightly after bathing hands in warm water. Passive ROM exercises to fingers daily. No pain reported by client with passive finger extension to full ROM during bath. Client not doing ROM exercises by self. Still needs assistance with ADL. Client was quite active in quilting club prior to admission, as well as being an active member of church group and maintaining her own apartment. Consultation with OT indicates sewing activities available. Client continues to remain in room by self most of day.

A. ROM exercises are helping finger extension. Client understands exercise regimen and its benefits but is not participating in this. May be having difficulty in adjusting to change in role, and status of being in nursing home. This could be indicated by lack of participation in activities and exercise regimen. Since client was an active and independent person prior to admission, she may see being in nursing home as taking on a "sick role" that she does not wish to assume.[1] Mobility in fingers present, and exercise needs to be encouraged before contractures form.

P. *Diagnostic:*

1. Talk with client at 2 P.M. today re her thoughts and feelings about being in nursing home, change of lifestyle. Will continue to spend time each day with client to talk about whatever concerns she wants to discuss.

Therapeutic:

1. Continue daily ROM exercises to fingers of both hands during bath. Follow bathing with lotion to hands and fingers—client to apply this.
2. Continue to assist with ADL. Utilize long shoehorn, elastic shoelaces so that client can assist self as much as possible.

Teaching and Referral:

1. Review with client availability of OT.
2. If client agrees, visit OT area with her and talk with therapist about sewing activities.
3. Review plan in 1 week → 11/20/75.

[1]The sick role, while allowing for care and protection, also involves loss of some freedom and autonomy. Pamela Holsclaw Mitchell, *Concepts Basic to Nursing,* McGraw-Hill, New York, 1977, p. 17.

DATE:

ASSESSMENT PRACTICE 20: Progress Notes

After writing and implementing your initial plan with a client, evaluate the effectiveness of the plan by writing a progress note.

Date: Time: Problem # and name:

S.

O.

A.

P. *Diagnostic:*

Therapeutic:

Teaching:

Referral:

UNIT 9

Assessment of Mobility/Comfort/Rest

OBJECTIVES

When you have completed this unit you should be able to:

1. Collect a data base for assessment of mobility/comfort/rest by interview, inspection, palpation, and consultation including:
   a. subjective (history) data
   b. objective (examination) data
2. Add to the client's problem list any actual, potential, or client-identified problems and/or health maintenance needs that emerge from the data base.
3. Write initial plans and begin nursing intervention.

HISTORY AND PHYSICAL EXAMINATION FOR MOBILITY/COMFORT/REST

Mobility is almost always affected by changes in a client's health status, and is an area where many nursing interventions can contribute to a client's well-being. These interventions include assisting clients with ambulating and with other activities of daily living such as eating or bathing, helping them maintain a normal range of joint motion, and preventing dysfunction resulting from disuse. Mobility assessment is important because the nurse needs to know what a client is able to do on his own before health maintenance and preventive and restorative intervention can be planned. Mobility assessment is equally important in helping the practitioner learn about how clients view themselves and their problems. Many people today consider their mobility a measure of their wellness or illness. For example, a client may state, "I really didn't think I needed to come to the clinic, but when I couldn't walk up the steps anymore, I decided I'd get some help." People may also consider mobility as a means of defining themselves and their roles, as, for example, the 45-year-old male client who had a myocardial infarction and whose response to prescribed bed rest was "I'm a busy person, I've got a family to support, I can't sit around in bed all day!" Activity and mobility patterns then provide significant data for the total assessment of the client.

Before you actually begin the examination part of the mobility assessment, you may need to learn or review the skill of performing joint range-of-motion exercises. Textbooks, articles, and audio-visual aids for basic nursing skills (some of which are listed in the bibliography for this chapter) can help you do this. These sources can also help you learn or review how to assist clients with ambulation and other mobility needs.

Beginning with this assessment, you must be more aware of the need to use good nursing judgment in order to perform assessments safely. In the case of mobility, for example, you must determine first whether there are any medical restrictions on a client's mobility. Temporary immobility is sometimes necessary. You would not, for example, ask a client who has a physician's order for "complete bed rest" to walk around his room so you can assess his ability to walk and stand. Nor would you move a joint beyond the point of resistance or pain without special instructions from a nurse expert, physician, or physical therapist. This does not mean that an inexperienced nurse should assume that other professionals have adequately weighed a client's need for rest against the potential problems of immobility. To help you learn under what conditions it is appropriate for you to carry out the assessments and nursing interventions independently, you will need to use your skill of consultation with more experienced nurses and/or other health professionals concerned with mobility problems, such as physical and occupational therapists, and physicians.

Comfort and rest are important needs that we all have: pain and sleep, which affect these needs, are possible problematic areas that you and your clients will often encounter. Assisting clients in obtaining adequate sleep and rest, or in obtaining relief from pain, are important nursing functions. These functions may involve providing physical comfort by giving a backrub, altering the environment by opening a window or turning on a night light, or talking with the client about what he is currently experiencing.

A client's sleep pattern, and his perception of and reaction to pain, will influence his activity, nutrition, responsiveness to people and environment, and reactions to stress. As you begin this assessment with your client, remember that how your client perceives his comfort and rest needs is very important; these are subjective experiences and each client will talk about a wide range of experience which is unique. Pain and discomfort can have physiological or psychological causes, or both, so that if you make observations about a client's discomfort, it is important to validate this with him. At times, conferring with family members or other staff about your client's comfort and rest patterns is helpful.

In Assessment Practices 21 and 22 you will find outlines for the data base for a mobility assessment. The purpose is to help you determine whether your client needs nursing assistance in mobility, comfort, and rest. You have already collected the additional data you will need to consider broader mobility problems, i.e., the activity pattern for the typical 24-hour day and other data in the client profile. Use these data and if necessary do some further interviewing to find out if your client's mobility is limited to one building or one block or an entire community, etc. Keep in mind the goal of discovering the meaning of mobility restrictions to the client; this knowledge will be valuable as you write plans for intervention.

SELECTED BIBLIOGRAPHY

Mobility, Comfort, and Rest Assessment

Bates, Barbara: *A Guide to Physical Examination,* J. B. Lippincott, Philadelphia, 1974, pp. 226-262, 299-300.

Cuica, Rudy, Jennie Bradish, and Suzanne M. Trombly: "Range of Motion Exercises, Active and Passive, a Handbook," *Nursing '73,* **3:**25-37, December 1973.

Fuerst, Elinor V., LuVerne Wolff, and Marlene H. Weitzel: *Fundamentals of Nursing,* 5th ed., J. B. Lippincott, Philadelphia, 1974, pp. 268-317.

Mitchell, Pamela Holsclaw: *Concepts Basic to Nursing,* McGraw-Hill, New York, 1977, pp. 291-337, 522-551.

Synder, Mariah, and Rebecca Baum: "Assessing Station and Gait," *American Journal of Nursing,* **74**:1256-1257, 1974.

Webb, Kenneth J.: "Early Assessment of Orthopedic Injuries," *American Journal of Nursing,* **74**:1048-1053, 1974.

DATE:

ASSESSMENT PRACTICE 21: Health History for Mobility/Comfort/Rest

History

1. *Mobility—Client's perception of the following:*
   a. Are there any medical restrictions on activity (physician's prescription for bed rest, bathroom privileges, etc.)?

   b. Are there any institutional restrictions on activity (when are visitors allowed, does the client have to have a pass if he wishes to go out for a few hours, are bedrails, restraints, used)?

   c. Are there any environmental restrictions on activity (what is available for physical exercise and activities, and what intellectual stimulation is available)?

   d. Does the client now have, or has he ever had in the past:

      (1) paralysis

      (2) weakness

      (3) contractures

      (4) abnormal movements (spasms, tremors, tics)

      (5) stiffness

      (6) trauma (accidents, injuries)

      (7) swelling, pain, or tenderness

      (8) difficulty with walking, reaching, or other movements

   e. Any aids used for ambulation—cane, crutches, walker, etc.?

f. Medications client is taking to aid mobility/activity. Include summary of client's understanding of medications.

How does the client describe the following?

2. *Sleep*
   a. Normal sleep pattern (number of hours, time, whether the client feels rested, naps).

   b. Any changes in sleep pattern—describe.

   c. Characteristics of sleep (sound, light, dreams, nightmares, restless, quiet).

   d. Aids used for sleep (beverages, positional comfort, reading, rituals, medications—sedatives, hypnotics).

3. *Comfort*
   a. Presence of pain or discomfort (onset, progression, duration, character, location, course, aggravating or relieving factors).

   b. Treatment to relieve pain or discomfort (prior to and during current experience—analgesics, positioning, exercise, compresses, talking about it).

DATE:

ASSESSMENT PRACTICE 22: Physical Examination for Mobility/Comfort/Rest

Physical Examination

1. *Mobility*
   a. general movements (smooth, jerky, tremor)

   b. handedness (right or left)

   c. range of joint motion (evaluate and record on chart following this assessment)

   d. ability to perform activities of daily living (evaluate and record on chart following this assessment)

   e. stance
      (1) posture when standing

      (2) need for support when standing (equilibrium, balance)

   f. gait
      (1) assistance needed for ambulation

      (2) posture when walking

      (3) observe for shuffling, limping, foot dragging, foot slapping, if arms swing freely

2. *Sleep*

As suggested earlier, if you are not present when client is sleeping, you may want to confer with family and/or staff members regarding client's sleep patterns, including naps. The Kardex and nurses' notes on the chart may also have information regarding sleep patterns.

3. *Comfort*
   a. indications of possible pain, or discomfort
      (1) restlessness, withdrawal, difficulty in sleeping, loss of appetite

      (2) increase in muscle tension

      (3) changes in physical structure (swelling, skin intactness-color-texture, trauma)

      (4) change in temperature, BP, respirations (see oxygenation assessment)

Laboratory Data

Include x-ray reports indicating joint abnormalities, bone deformities, fractures.

Medications Related to Mobility/Comfort/Rest

Such medications include stimulants, skeletal muscle relaxants, analgesics, tranquilizers. Include the same data for reviewing medications pertaining to mobility as you utilized in reviewing medications in the physical structure assessment.

Assessment of Range of Joint Motion

First determine which motions can be performed actively without assistance by the client, then assess passive range of motion for joints which cannot be moved through the full normal range actively.

F = full motion; P = partial motion; 0 = no motion

Specify motion in degrees if possible.

Joints	Motions	Observed Motions			
		Active		Passive	
Neck	flexion				
	extension				
	rotation				
Trunk	flexion				
	extension				
		Right	Left	Right	Left
Shoulder	flexion				
	extension				
	abduction				
	adduction				
	int. rotation				
	ext. rotation				
Elbow	flexion				
	suppination				
	pronation				
Wrist	flexion				
	extension				
	ul. deviation				
	ra. deviation				
Fingers	flexion				
	extension				
Thumb	flexion				
	extension				
Hip	flexion				
	extension				
	abduction				
	adduction				
	int. rotation				
	ext. rotation				
Knee	flexion				
	extension				
Ankle	flexion				
	extension				
	inversion				
	eversion				
Toes	flexion				
	extension				

Assessment for Activities of Daily Living

Grade only activities actually observed as follows:

G = good, independent and at least fairly efficient
F = fair, very slow, insecure, or tiring
P = partial, requires supervision or some assistance
O = zero, not even partial performance possible

Hygiene		**Locomotion**	
Brush, comb hair		Chair, sitting down	
Brush teeth		Chair, getting up	
Wash hands		Room walking	
Wash face		Stairs up	
Wash feet		Stairs down	
Turn faucet		Walk, turn corner	
Take shower		Walk to bathroom	
Take bath (tub)		Get into car	
Use handkerchief			
Eating		**Writing, Reading**	
Eat with Spoon		Write by hand	
Eat with fork		Use typewriter	
Use knife		Unfold newspaper	
Butter bread		Hold book	
Drink-glass, cup		Turn pages	
Dressing		**Miscellaneous**	
Undershirt, bra		Doorknob	
Shorts, panties		Use drawer	
Shirt, blouse		Dial telephone	
Trousers, skirt		Use scissors	
Socks, stockings		Use keys	
Slip on Shoes		Move chair	
Tie laces		Count coins	
Jacket, dress			
Zipper, buttons			

Source: Adapted from and used with permission of Armour Pharmaceuticals, "Evaluation Chart: Activities of Daily Living."

DATE:

ASSESSMENT PRACTICE 23: Initial Plan

After reviewing your data on mobility/comfort/rest, identify any new problems and record them on the client's problem list. Remember that this problem list is the "table of contents" for the POHR. It is the first page of the POHR and all problems with which the health team are working are listed here, whether old, current, or new. If you have identified any new problems and/or health maintenance needs from this assessment, you will want to write initial plans for them. The initial plan outline is listed below. You may wish to refer back to Unit 7 for guidelines in writing plans. At the end of each of the succeeding units in this workbook you will find an outline for an initial plan. As you proceed with the assessments you will be adding more problems to the original problem list and writing additional plans.

Initial Plan

Date: Time: Problem # and name:

S.

O.

A.

P. *Diagnostic:*

Therapeutic:

Teaching:

Referral:

UNIT 10

Oxygenation Assessment

OBJECTIVES

When you have completed this unit you should be able to:

1. Collect a data base for assessment of oxygenation by interview, inspection, palpation, auscultation, and consultation including:
   a. subjective (history) data
   b. objective (examination, laboratory, chart) data
2. Discuss the rationale for explaining nursing procedures to clients and the need for client collaboration in such procedures.
3. Utilize progress notes to monitor and review problems and nursing care.

HISTORY AND PHYSICAL EXAMINATION FOR OXYGENATION

At this point you have already worked with your client(s) in assessing physical structure and mobility/comfort/rest patterns. You have utilized your interviewing skills in history taking and have utilized the physical assessment skills of inspection and palpation. In the following assessment of the oxygenation status of your client you will be adding to these skills the skill of auscultation to help you in collecting data. Accurate history taking continues to be of the greatest importance. Clients usually are able to offer much information about their heart and breathing status; to most of us these functions are indeed seen as vital to our health. Again, use of open-ended questions/statements such as "Do you have any difficulties now, (or did you in the past), with breathing (heart trouble, anemia)?" "Tell me more about that," are helpful to aid the client in describing how he sees this area of his health. If possible, the client should be encouraged to give his impressions of any limitations and/or impairments in this area that seem to affect his everyday living. This information is essential in planning nursing care. For example:

Client: I get out of breath climbing up stairs. I guess I have to expect this—I'm 82 years old.

Nurse: Do you have to climb stairs very often?

Client: I live in a fifth-floor walk-up apartment. Sometimes I run out of food but I don't go to the store because it's just too hard to get up and down those stairs more than a couple of times a week.

This conversation reveals many needs that require consideration in planning care—nutrition and mobility needs as well as oxygenation needs.

Your history and physical assessment of the client's oxygenation status should include data on circulation, respiration, and temperature. Your physical assessment skills of inspection, palpation, and auscultation provide direct and indirect data about the functioning of the heart, lungs, blood vessels, and blood. It would be helpful to review the normal anatomy and physiology of these areas before beginning your assessment so that you may compare your findings with normal values.

Since you will be using some specific tools in addition to your own senses and resources in this assessment, i.e., stethoscope, sphygmomanometer, thermometer, it is important to explain to your client what you plan to do beforehand. The client's positive participation and cooperation in many parts of the procedure are essential for his sense of safety and security as well as for the accurate performance of the procedure. Performing the procedure and recording results must be done accurately. You record what you observe or hear. If in doubt, for example, about where you first hear the systolic sound in taking a blood pressure, consult with your instructor or a professional staff member.

Laboratory data provides much information about your client's oxygenation status. In checking your client's record, read the most current lab data (check the date). You may also wish to refer back to previous reports and see if there have been any significant changes.

Before beginning the actual physical assessment of your client's oxygenation status, you will want to make a general statement of your overall observations. General observations pertaining to oxygenation status could include:

Appearance-older or younger than stated age?
Over or under weight?
Postural interferences to respiration?
Oriented or confused?
Irritable, anxious?
Color of skin, lips, nails?
Intactness of skin, rashes?
Environmental temperature and humidity?

Physical assessment for this pattern will include the skills of inspection, palpation, and auscultation. The cephalocaudal approach will guide your assessment of circulatory, respiratory, and temperature status.

SELECTED BIBLIOGRAPHY

Oxygenation Assessment

Bates, Barbara: *A Guide to Physical Examination,* J. B. Lippincott, Philadelphia, 1974, pp. 73-81, 99-102, 112-113, 137-140.

Brown, Marie Scott, and Mary M. Alexander: "Physical Examination, Part 11, Examining the Heart," *Nursing '74,* **4**:41-47, November 1974.

——, and ——: "Physical Examination, Part 12, Examining the Chest and Lungs," *Nursing '75,* **5**:44-48, January 1975.

Delaney, Mary T.: "Examining the Chest, Part 1, The Lungs," *Nursing '75,* **5**:12-14, August 1975.

——: "Examining the Chest, Part 2, The Heart," *Nursing '75,* **5**:41-46, September 1975.

Fuerst, Elinor V., LuVerne Wolff, and Marlene H. Weitzel: *Fundamentals of Nursing,* 5th ed., J. B. Lippincott, Philadelphia, 1974, pp. 214-226, 396-415.

Gordon, Marjory: "Assessing Activity Tolerance," *American Journal of Nursing,* **76**:72-75, 1976.

Mitchell, Pamela Holsclaw: *Concepts Basic to Nursing,* McGraw-Hill, New York, 1977, pp. 392-398, 437-491.

Sparks, Colleen: "Peripheral Pulses," *American Journal of Nursing,* **75**:1132-1133, 1975.

DATE:

ASSESSMENT PRACTICE 24: Health History for Oxygenation

History

1. *Respiratory*

   a. Does the client now have, or has he ever had in the past:

   chest pain

   cough (productive, chronic, acute, time of day, with activity)

   expectoration (color, amount, odor, viscosity, hemoptysis)

   dyspnea

   orthopnea

   wheezing, noisy breathing, snoring

   frequent colds

   b. Does the client use any supportive devices for breathing (nebulizers, humidifiers, respirators)

   c. Does the client use any medications that affect respiratory status?

   d. What are the client's impressions of impairment and limitations, if any, of respiratory status on daily life (activities, sleep, habits)?

   e. If client experiences anxiety or apprehension, does he see this as affecting breathing? If so, describe.

2. *Circulatory:*

a. Does the client now have, or has he ever had in the past:

heart disease

chest or epigastric pain

palpitation

fatigue

heart murmur

problems with blood pressure

cyanosis

edema

cold extremities

pains in legs when walking

anemia

bruising

b. What are the client's impressions of impairment and limitations, if any, of circulatory status on daily life (sleep, activities, habits)?

c. Is the client taking any medications that affect circulatory status?

3. *Temperature status*

Give client's description of:

a. feelings of warmth and cold

b. usual measures for temperature comfort

c. perspiration (presence, absence, pattern, night sweats)

d. environmental temperature and humidty

e. use of medications that affect temperature status

DATE:

ASSESSMENT PRACTICE 25: Physical Examination for Oxygenation

Physical Examination

	Rate	Quality	Rhythm
1. *Head*			
a. R temporal pulse			
L temporal pulse			

	R	L
b. eyes		
(1) sclera (color)		
(2) conjunctiva (color)		

c. nose
   (1) deviation

   (2) breathing through nose

d. mouth
   (1) color of lips, mucous membrane

   (2) patency of airway (clear, obstructed)

	Rate	Quality	Rhythm
2. *Neck*			
a. R carotid pulse			
b. L carotid pulse			

3. *Chest*
   a. size and shape (ratio of anteroposterior diameter to lateral diameter)

b. respirations

(1) rate, rhythm, depth, ease, noise

(2) change in relation to activity level, position, emotion, pain, humidity, air pollution

(3) ventilatory motion (abdominal, thoracic)

(4) sternal retractions

(5) cough, wheezing

4. *Apical impulse* Rate Quality Rhythm

5. *Back (contour and postural influences on respiration—kyphosis, lordosis)*

6. *Arms* Rate Quality Rhythm

a. R brachial pulse

b. L brachial pulse

c. R radial pulse

d. L radial pulse

e. pulse deficit (apical rate—radial rate)

f. pulse response in relation to activity level, anxiety, pain

g. skin temperature, color

h. nails

(1) color

(2) clubbing

i. blood pressure Systolic/muffling/diastolic

(1) R arm sitting

(2) L arm sitting

(3) R arm lying

(4) L arm lying

(5) pulse pressure

7. *Buttocks (sacral edema)*

8. *Legs*

a. skin color, temperature

b. pulses	Rate	Quality	Rhythm
(1) R femoral			
(2) L femoral			
(3) R popliteal			
(4) L popliteal			
(5) R dorsalis pedis			
(6) L dorsalis pedis			
(7) R posterior tibial			
(8) L posterior tibial			

c. edema (extent, location)

9. *Body temperature (measure with thermometer)*
   a. oral

   b. rectal

   c. axillary

10. *Exercise tolerance (change in vital signs, amount of activity tolerated)*

Laboratory Data[1]

1. Respiratory—chest x ray, skin test, blood gas analysis—PO_2, PCO_2, blood pH

2. Circulatory—chest x ray, hemoglobin, hematocrit

Medications Related to Respiratory, Circulatory, Temperature Status

1. A classification of medications affecting respiratory status includes bronchodilators, antibiotics, antitussives, expectorants, nasal decongestants.

2. A classification of medications affecting circulatory status includes vasodilators, antihypertensives, vasoconstrictors, cardiac glycosides, antianemic drugs, anticoagulent drugs, and antiarrhythmic drugs.

3. A classification of medication affecting temperature status includes an antipyretic.

[1]Some of these values may be entered on the Health Maintenance Flow Sheet, page 67.

DATE:

ASSESSMENT PRACTICE 26: Initial Plan

Initial Plan

Date: Time: Problem # and name:

S.

O.

A.

P. *Diagnostic:*

Therapeutic:

Teaching:

Referral:

DATE:

ASSESSMENT PRACTICE 27: Progress Note

You have at this point completed three assessments, (1) physical structure, (2) mobility/comfort/rest, and (3) oxygenation, as well as the client profile, and have identified problems and initiated plans. If you have not already done so, you may now wish to look at the problems and plans that need to be reviewed in terms of current status, additional new data, effectiveness of nursing intervention, and how the client is viewing what is happening to him. As discussed in Unit 8, the above factors are reviewed and evaluated by the use of a progress note. The outline for writing a progress note is given below. Progress note outlines will be presented at the end of each of the succeeding units to assist you in your ongoing review of initial plans and problems.

Progress Notes

Date: Time: Problem # and name:

S.

O.

A.

P. *Diagnostic:*

Therapeutic:

Teaching:

Referral:

UNIT 11

Nutrition/Elimination Assessment

OBJECTIVES

When you have completed this unit you should be able to:

1. Collect a data base for assessment of nutrition/elimination by interview, inspection, palpation, and consultation including:
   a. subjective (history) data
   b. objective (examination, laboratory, chart) data
2. Evaluate the adequacy of a client's nutritional intake in terms of the basic food groups.
3. Evaluate a client's fluid balance in terms of client's needs and intake and output.

HISTORY AND PHYSICAL EXAMINATION FOR NUTRITION/ELIMINATION

Whether or not we agree in total with the common saying, "you are what you eat," we probably all would agree that nutrition does contribute a great deal to a person's health. Nurses are involved in working with clients and their nutritional needs in all stages of health and illness as well as in prevention. You may work with an expectant mother in planning her prenatal diet, following through on possible diet changes after she has delivered, and then planning with her the new baby's diet. You may work with an adolescent boy who has just been diagnosed as a diabetic and who needs some help in adjusting his diet needs to this new illness. You might also be working with an elderly woman living alone on a monthly social security check who cannot afford to pay her rent bills if she buys appropriate food for her nutritional needs. However, before beginning to work with a client in the area of nutrition, it is important to inquire about his eating patterns and habits, his likes and dislikes, and to learn about the physical, social, cultural, and symbolic aspects of food and eating that influence his nutrition. This also applies to your history taking of fluid balance and of elimination. At times some beginning practitioners may feel uncomfortable about asking a client about his habits of elimination. This is understandable, since people in our society do not routinely discuss this part of their health. It is helpful to remember that if you have established an open, honest, interested, and caring climate in your interviews, most people will readily answer your questions. As in previous assessments, you may wish to consult with family members about a client's particular eating habits and food preferences; this would be important, for example, if your client were a small child, or an acutely ill person. If your client is in an institution, a dietician or other staff member might be consulted. You might also be interested in learning about community agencies that are involved in the area of nutrition, such as Weight Watchers, or consumers' bureaus. In some communities, clients who have had surgery that affects elimination status have organized "ostomy" clubs.

Before making any initial plans for your client's nutrition, it is important that you evaluate the adequacy of your client's diet in terms of the basic four food groups: (1) meats, fish, and poultry; (2) fruits and vegetables; (3) milk and other dairy products; and (4) bread and other cereals. You must also learn what your client thinks about his diet. The history data outline in Assessment Practice 28 will help you with this. In some instances, it may be important to keep an accurate record of a client's fluid balance. This is known as an intake and output record. You and/or the client will need to accurately measure all fluids taken in and eliminated. You may wish to review the part of the metric system that relates to fluid measure; for example, how many cubic centimeters (ccs) are in a 12-oz can of soda?

Before you start your physical assessment, observe and record the general appearance of your client in regard to nutrition. Does she appear overweight? What about fat distribution—is one side of her body heavier than the other, is the upper part of her body heavier than the lower, is she "skin and bones?" What is the general appearance of skin, hair, and nails? As you start your physical assessment, you may find that you have already collected some of the data if you have worked with the client previously. If so, it is not necessary to repeat that particular area of assessment; you may refer back to the earlier data.

Example: Hair (see physical structure assessment of 10/12/75)

Charts, Kardex, and members of the health team are resources for additional pertinent data.

SELECTED BIBLIOGRAPHY

Nutrition, Elimination, Fluid Balance Assessment

Bates, Barbara: *A Guide To Physical Examination,* J. B. Lippincott, Philadelphia, 1974, pp. 27, 158-160, 171-172.

Brown, Marie Scott, and Mary Alexander: "Physical Examination, Part 10, Examining Mouth and Throat," *Nursing'74,* **4**:57-61, August 1974.

Fuerst, Elinor V., LuVerne Wolff, and Marlene H. Weitzel: *Fundamentals of Nursing,* 5th ed., J. B. Lippincott, Philadelphia, 1974, pp. 318-395.

Mitchell, Pamela Holsclaw: *Concepts Basic to Nursing,* McGraw-Hill, New York, 1977, pp. 339-391, 398-435.

Willacker, Jean: "Bowel Sounds," *American Journal of Nursing,* **73**:2100-2101, 1973.

"Examination of the Abdomen," Programmed Instruction, *American Journal of Nursing,* **74**:1679-1700, 1974.

DATE:

ASSESSMENT PRACTICE 28: Health History for Nutrition/Elimination

History

1. *Nutrition*
   a. appetite

   b. usual eating patterns and usual times (use chart following this history section)

   c. eating behavior (gulper, nibbler, eat-and-run, fast-and-feast)

   d. food likes and dislikes

   e. food restrictions (culture, religion, allergies, food intolerance—describe)

   f. changes in pattern (special diet, appetite changes, stress)

   g. assistance needed in eating

   h. diet supplements (preparations such as sustagen, vitamins)

   i. weight gain or loss (steady, sporadic, over what period of time)

   j. symbolic meaning of food (socialization, love, reward, eat when nervous)

   k. past or present experiences of
      (1) diabetes

      (2) nutritional disease

      (3) flatulence

(4) burping

(5) nausea, vomiting

(6) heartburn

(7) pain

(8) difficulty in swallowing, tasting

l. artificial means of food intake (tube feeding, hyperalimentation)

m. usual care of teeth (daily, dentist's visits; if dentures, type, fit, effectiveness)

n. use of any medications affecting metabolism, digestion of foods, nutritional status

2. *Fluid balance*

a. pattern of fluid intake (amount in 24 h, types preferred)

b. changes in fluid intake (related to health problem, increase or decrease)

c. past or present experiences of

(1) thirst

(2) weight gain or loss

(3) edema

(4) neuromuscular weakness or irritability

3. *Pattern of fluid elimination*

a. sweating (times, amount)

b. urination (frequency, urgency, pain, burning, dribbling, nocturia)

c. urine (amount, color, odor, unusual constituents)

d. method of elimination (toilet, bedpan, commode, urinal, needs assistance)

e. continence/incontinence (circumstances, ways of coping)

f. changes in usual pattern—describe

g. drainage from wounds

h. use of any medication affecting fluid balance and/or elimination

4. *Pattern of bowel elimination*
   a. usual pattern (frequency, time of day, aids normally used—beverages, exercises, enemas)

   b. character of stool (color, amount, odor, consistency, unusual constituents)

   c. diarrhea, constipation (acute, chronic)

   d. continence/incontinence (circumstances, ways of coping)

   e. changes in usual pattern—describe

   f. hemorrhoids

   g. artificial orifices for elimination (ileal conduit—urine, colostomy—bowel, client's way of caring for this).

24-HOUR NUTRITION SUMMARY

For each meal and/or snack, record the food, its amount, and how it was prepared, under the appropriate column. A peanut butter and jelly sandwich, for example, might be recorded as 2 slices white bread under the "bread and cereals" column, 2 tablespoons peanut butter and 1 tablespoon jelly under the condiments column along with the time and place where it was consumed. Another example would be a broiled chicken leg prepared without salt eaten at 5 p.m. at the hospital cafeteria recorded under the "meats, fish, and poultry" column.

Meal or Snack	Meats, Fish and Poultry	Fruits and Vegetables	Milk and Dairy Products	Bread and Cereals	**Other** (condiments such as salt, salad dressing, gravy; soft drinks and alcoholic beverages, etc.)
Breakfast Time ______ Place ______					
Lunch Time ______ Place ______					
Dinner Time ______ Place ______					
Other (Snacks, Supplements) Time ______ Place ______					
	Evaluation of Adequacy: Evaluate the nutritional adequacy of your client's food intake in each of the above categories, using the "basic four" requirements.				

DATE:

ASSESSMENT PRACTICE 29: Physical Examination for Nutrition/Elimination

Physical Examination[2]

1. *Height and weight (metric system)*

2. *Head*
   a. level of consciousness

   b. hair (texture, sheen, distribution)

   c. skin (texture, dryness, turgor)

   d. mouth
      (1) mucous membranes (intactness, dry, moist, color, presence of debris, crusts, lesions)

      (2) breath

      (3) teeth (dentulous, edentulous, condition)

      (4) gums (color, condition)

      (5) tongue (dry, presence of crust, debris)

3. *Throat*
   a. exudate, injection

   b. ability to swallow

[2]*Note:* If you have already recorded this data in previous assessments, refer to those assessments rather than repeating the description here.

4. *Abdomen*
   a. contour

   b. bowel sounds

5. *Rectum*
   a. hemorrhoids

   b. fissures

6. *Arms and hands*
   a. skin (texture, dryness, turgor)

   b. ability to feed self

7. *Legs and feet*
   a. skin (texture, dryness, turgor)

   b. edema (pattern and location, extent)

8. *Intake and output*
   Obtain a 24-hour record of your client's I & O and record, using metric liquid measure. Your client, if able, may help you by keeping a record of this also. Evaluate I & O in terms of adequacy and meeting client's needs.

9. *Urine*
   color, clear or cloudy, odor, unusual constituents—compare with normal values

10. *Stool*
    color, form, odor, consistency, unusual constituents—compare with normal values

Laboratory Data

1. *Electrolytes*[3] Normal values

2. *Blood sugar*[3] Normal values

3. *Urine*[3] Normal values
   a. color

   b. pH

   c. specific gravity

   d. sugar and acetone

   e. WBC

4. *Stool* Normal values
   a. eggs/parasites

   b. occult blood

Medications Related to Nutrition/Elimination/Fluid Balance

(Objective data-from Kardex, chart, M.D.'s order sheet)

1. A classification of medications affecting metabolism and digestion of foods and nutritional status includes minerals, vitamins, hormones, antacids, antiemetics.

2. A classification of medications affecting fluid balance and elimination includes diuretics, hormones, drugs acting on bladder, urinary antiseptics.

3. A classification of medications affecting bowel elimination includes cathartics, antidiarrheics, stool softeners.

[3]Some of these values may be entered on the Health Maintenance Flow Sheet on page 67.

DATE:

ASSESSMENT PRACTICE 30: Initial Plan

Initial Plan

Date: Time: Problem # and Name

S.

O.

A.

P. *Diagnostic:*

Therapeutic:

Teaching:

Referral:

DATE:

ASSESSMENT PRACTICE 31: Progress Note

Progress Note

Date: Time: Problem # and name:

S.

O.

A.

P. *Diagnostic:*

Therapeutic:

Teaching:

Referral:

UNIT 12

Mental / Emotional Status Assessment

OBJECTIVES

When you have completed this unit you should be able to:

1. Assess, by interviewing, inspection, and consultation, your client's mental/emotional status.
2. Describe how your client perceives himself as a person and how he perceives his interpersonal relationships.
3. Assess your client's use of defense mechanisms.

HISTORY AND EXAMINATION FOR MENTAL/EMOTIONAL STATUS

Perhaps in no other assessment area are your interviewing skills and ability to listen as important as in the assessment of your client's mental/emotional status. It is important that you help your client feel that you are interested in him, and accept him. He must feel assured that you will not judge what he tells you about himself "right" or "wrong" or "good" or "bad," and that you care about him as a person. This doesn't mean that you have to agree with everything your client tells you, for indeed you may not. However, what can develop is that you and your client come to trust each other with the sharing of information in spite of any differences in lifestyles and values.

A major purpose of the mental/emotional status assessment is to learn how the client perceives and feels about himself. How does he see himself relating to others, and vice versa, and how does he see himself coping with everyday living and stress? How people view themselves includes how they see themselves in their roles as men or women —breadwinner, homemaker, compliant, assertive, parent, single person—how they view their sexual identity, and what their preferences are in choosing sexual partners. As mentioned in the previous unit on interviewing it may be difficult at times for both beginning and experienced practitioners to ask questions of clients that involve personal matters not always discussed openly in our society. How people really feel about themselves, sexuality, and the wish to hurt themselves or someone else are examples of such personal matters. Again, it is important to remember that if clients feel accepted for whom they are without being judged, they usually will feel able to talk about themselves. Often clients experience a sense of relief when the nurse asks a question about their sexuality, for example, or about a fear they have expressed, because a topic of possible concern is being explored by someone who seems to think this is important and not unusual to discuss.

Another major purpose of the mental/emotional status assessment is for you to observe how your client is functioning and to evaluate this in relation to his own perceptions. For example, you will be assessing your client's behavior, mood, speech, reality orientation, and thought processes and content. You will also want to assess the defense mechanisms your client is utilizing (remember that we all use these mechanisms daily to cope) and the developmental level that your client has reached.

The primary tool you will be using in the history and examination of this assessment is yourself. Your ability to observe, to listen, to know whether to ask a question or to be silent are some of the creative uses of yourself that will assist the client to learn about himself and his concerns. They will also enable you to make a more accurate assessment and to plan nursing care.

SELECTED BIBLIOGRAPHY

Mental/Emotional Assessment

Bates, Barbara: *A Guide to Physical Examination,* J. B. Lippincott, 1974, pp. 306-313.

Mackinnon, Roger A., and Robert Michels: *The Psychiatric Interview in Clinical Practice,* W. B. Saunders, Philadelphia, 1971, pp. 3-64.

Mitchell, Pamela Holsclaw: *Concepts Basic to Nursing,* McGraw-Hill, New York, 1977, pp. 189-241.

Prior, John A., and Jack S. Silberstein: *Physical Diagnosis,* C. V. Mosby, 1973, pp. 29-47.

"Understanding Defense Mechanisms," Programmed Instruction, *American Journal of Nursing,* **72,** September 1972.

DATE:

ASSESSMENT PRACTICE 32: Health History for Mental/ Emotional Status

History

1. Client's perception and understanding of his health problem(s) and goals of medical and nursing therapy.

2. Beliefs and attitudes about illness (sickness as punishment).

3. Previous experience with, and reaction to, illness and/or hospitalization.

4. Client's description of himself; how does he see himself as a person?

    a. general mood and emotional responses

    b. role played or assigned in family, community

    c. concept of self (sense of worth, self-esteem)

    d. reactions to stress and ways of coping with stressful situations.

    e. patterns of relating to others

f. sexuality
   (1) sexual preference (heterosexual, homosexual)

   (2) pleasure/discomfort

   (3) responsiveness

g. special concerns or fears

5. Client's perception of reality orientation—time, place, month, year.

6. Client's perception of memory—remote and recent.

7. Has client ever had a wish to die or to harm anyone else? Has anyone in his family attempted suicide or violent behavior?

   a. History of attempts, plans, intent to carry out plan.

   b. Has client experienced a recent loss? Are there other provoking factors?

8. Has client sensed changes in behavior, perception, thought process, mood, anxiety, body functioning, or changes in any of the above areas?

9. Is client using any substances that alter his emotional responses? (Include prescribed drugs such as tranquilizers, sedatives, antidepressants, amphetamines; "street" drugs such as marijuana, LSD; over-the-counter drugs; alcoholic beverages; coffee, tea, and cola beverages containing caffeine.)

DATE:

ASSESSMENT PRACTICE 33: Examination for Mental/Emotional Status

Examination

1. *Overall impression*
   Briefly write your general impression of your client, including apparent physical condition, general health, approximate height and weight, posture, eye contact, appropriateness of dress for age-sex-season-setting, and relatedness to you as the interviewer.

2. *Degree of reality orientation*
   a. knowledge of time-place-month-year

   b. memory—remote and recent

3. *Intellectual development relative to age*
   (estimate normal, above- or below-average intelligence, mental retardation)

4. *Behavior*
   a. motor activity (unusual movements, over- or under-active)

   b. awareness of environment

5. *Speech*
   a. sound (loud, soft, monotonic)

   b. rate

6. *Emotional expression (mood or affect)*
   a. appropriateness to topic being discussed

   b. overall impression of mood/affect

7. *Thought processes*
   a. quality of responses—appropriate or inappropriate

   b. ability to understand and follow directions

   c. attention span

   d. spontaneity, flexibility/rigidity

   e. connections between ideas

Thought content
   a. central themes (what client talks about)

   b. special preoccupations (hallucinations, delusions, phobias, obsessive thoughts, compulsive behaviors)

   c. extent to which special concerns or fears interfere with client's functioning

   d. thoughts of hurting self or others and evaluation of risk (past attempts, self or family, existence of plans, intent, history of recent loss).

9. *Ways of coping with stressful situations*
   use of defense mechanisms, "fight or flight"

10. *Ego strengths*
   a. judgment (how to budget money, plan activities, dress appropriately)

   b. sense of reality of world and self (realistic perception of self and environment)

   c. regulation and control of drives and impulses (pattern of planned versus impulsive behavior)

   d. ability to relate to others

   e. functional abilities, such as in work, at school, homemaking, parenting

Laboratory Data

1. EEG findings

2. Consider also normal and abnormal findings from other assessment areas since mental/emotional status affects and is affected by physical health.

Medications that Affect Mental/Emotional Status

A classification of medications affecting mental/emotional status includes major and minor tranquilizers, antidepressants, hallucinogenic drugs, sedatives, and amphetamines.

DATE:

ASSESSMENT PRACTICE 34: Initial Plan

Initial Plan

Date: Time: Problem # and name

S.

O.

A.

P. *Diagnostic:*

Therapeutic:

Teaching:

Referral:

DATE:

ASSESSMENT PRACTICE 35: Progress Note

Progress Note

Date: Time: Problem # and name

S.

O.

A.

P. *Diagnostic:*

Therapeutic:

Teaching:

Referral:

UNIT 13

Sensory Assessment

OBJECTIVES

When you have completed this unit, you should be able to:

1. Describe some simple tests for vision, hearing, speech, touch and temperature sensitivity, and proprioception.
2. Use the techniques described in this unit to perform a sensory assessment.

HISTORY AND PHYSICAL EXAMINATION FOR SENSORY ASSESSMENT

In evaluating your client's sensory status, you will be concerned with what are called the "special senses"—vision, hearing, taste, touch, and smell—and with proprioception (position sense). Each of these senses is unique and valuable both for safety and for the enjoyment of life. People can and do adjust to loss or absence of one or more of these senses, but nursing intervention is often an important factor in achieving this adaptation. Evaluating the environmental stimulation available to a retarded child, allowing a blind client to "feel" his way around a new hospital environment, and speaking distinctly and in short phrases or sentences to aid a deaf client's lipreading are examples of ways nurses assess and utilize data about a client's sensory status.

Accurate sensory examination depends on the client's ability and willingness to cooperate in the testing techniques. The nurse must fully understand the techniques in order to explain to the client what is expected and to adapt the assessment according to the client's ability to respond. For example, the nurse might be able to test the vision of a person who could not name the letters on a Snellen chart by using a special chart designed for children where the person only needs to indicate which way the E's point. Sometimes a practice or demonstration trial will help the client to give more accurate responses during the examination. If you or the client become fatigued, it is better to defer the examination to a later time to avoid inaccurate results. Remember, too, that sensory assessment is not complete without an evaluation of the client's sensory environment as well as his ability to receive, interpret, and respond to the stimuli around him.

To perform the sensory assessment you will need the following equipment: Snellen eye chart, small flashlight, cotton applicator sticks, cotton balls, a sterile safety pin, a ticking watch, test tubes of warm and cold water, and a few small common objects such as a comb, a watch, and a pencil. If you plan to perform Weber and Rinne hearing tests, you will also need a tuning fork.

This assessment is part of a complete neurological examination, which involves evaluation of motor functioning and perceptual abilities as well as sensory assessment. In the sensory assessment outline that follows, the starred items indicate additional data that would be included in a more complete examination. Data listed under other assessments in this workbook are also collected in a complete neurological examination, for example, data on gait, balance, involuntary movements, level of consciousness, ability to swallow, symmetry of eyelids.

SELECTED BIBLIOGRAPHY

Sensory Assessment

Alexander, Mary, and Marie Scott Brown: "Physical Examination, Part 8, Hearing Acuity," *Nursing '74,* **4**:61-65, April 1974.

Bates, Barbara: *A Guide to Physical Examination,* J. B. Lippincott, Philadelphia, 1974, pp. 284-285.

Brown, Marie Scott, and Mary Alexander: "Physical Examination, Part 5, The Eye," *Nursing '73,* **3**:41-49, December 1973.

____, and ____: "Physical Examination, Part 7, The Ear," *Nursing '74,* **4**:48-53, February 1974.

Erickson, Roberta: "Cranial Check, A Basic Neurological Assessment," *Nursing '74,* **4**:67-72, August 1974.

Fernsebner, Wilhemina: "Early Diagnosis of Acute Angle-Closure Glaucoma," *American Journal of Nursing,* **75**:1154-1155, July 1975.

Fuerst, Elinor V., LuVerne Wolff, and Marlene H. Weitzel, *Fundamentals of Nursing,* J. B. Lippincott, Philadelphia, 1974, pp. 475-482.

Hiles, David A.: "Strabismus," *American Journal of Nursing,* **74**:1082-1089, 1974.

Kahn, Howard: "Visual Dysfunctions—Some Easy Tests for Detecting Them in Children," *Nursing '74,* **4**:26-27, October 1974.

Mitchell, Pamela Holsclaw: *Concepts Basic to Nursing,* McGraw-Hill, New York, 1977, pp. 257-289.

Prior, John A., and Jack S. Silberstein, *Physical Diagnosis,* C. V. Mosby, St. Louis, 1973, pp. 349-392.

Sherman, Jacques L., and Sylvia Kleiman Fields, *Guide to Patient Evaluation,* Medical Examination Publishing, Flushing, N.Y., 1974, pp. 72-84, 95-96, 208-210.

"Patient Assessment: Examination of the Eye," Programmed Instruction, *American Journal of Nursing,* **75**, March 1975.

"Patient Assessment: Examination of the Eye," Programmed Instruction, Part I, *American Journal of Nursing,* **74**, November 1974.

"Patient Assessment: Examination of the Eye," Programmed Instruction, Part II, *American Journal of Nursing,* **75**, January 1975.

"Patient Assessment: Neurological Examination," Programmed Instruction, Part I, *American Journal of Nursing,* **75**, September 1975.

"Patient Assessment: Neurological Examination," Programmed Instruction, Part II, *American Journal of Nursing,* **75**, November 1975.

"Patient Assessment: Neurological Examination," Programmed Instruction, Part III, *American Journal of Nursing,* **76**, April 1976.

DATE:

ASSESSMENT PRACTICE 36: Sensory History

Enter dates for previous vision and hearing testing on Health Maintenance Flow Sheet.

1. *Eyes*
   a. how client evaluates own vision

   b. corrective lenses used

   c. any known vision problems

   d. extent to which problems interfere with ADL

   e. any diplopia, blurring, photophobia, color blindness, squinting, strabismus

   f. pain

   g. any other eye problems or recent changes in any of the above

2. *Ears*
   a. how client evaluates own hearing

   b. any infections, dizziness, tinnitis, pain

   c. known hearing problems

   d. extent to which problems interfere with ADL

   e. use of hearing aid, ability to lipread, or other ways of compensating for loss

   f. any other ear problems or recent changes in any of the above

3. *Nose*

a. client's evaluation of sense of smell

b. any known problems, such as nosebleeds, sinus problems, hayfever

4. *Mouth*

a. client's evaluation of sense of taste

b. review Nutrition/Elimination Assessment for additional relevant data

5. *Touch*

a. ability to feel heat, cold, pain, vibration

b. any other problems of touch (parasthesias, heightened sensitivity to touch)

6. *Sensory environment*

Note client's description of quality and quantity and appropriateness of environmental stimuli. What is client's preferred level of environmental stimulation (high, moderate, low)?

DATE:

ASSESSMENT PRACTICE 37: Sensory Examination

1. *Eyes*
   a. visual acuity (use Snellen chart)

      R eye

      L eye

      both eyes

   b. pupils

	R	L
pupils equal?		
pupils round?		
response to light		
response to accommodation		

   *extra ocular movements, visual fields

2. *Ears*

	R	L
a. hears ticking watch (at what distance)		
b. hears spoken voice (at what distance)		
c. hears whispered voice (at what distance)		
d. *Weber test		
*Rinne test		

*These items indicate additional data which would be included in a more complete examination.

3. *Speech*

   a. Evaluate conversational speech for fluency, hesitation, pronunciation. If any difficulty is suspected, test client's ability to repeat words, phrases, sentences; ask client to name two or three common objects (comb, watch, pencil).

   b. Record client's ability to follow simple directions (squeeze my hand, give me the pencil). If client has difficulty following spoken directions, try using gestures or written words.

4. *Smell*

   Beginning-level examinations usually do not include testing smell. If a problem is reported in the history, you could perform a simple test by asking client to close his eyes and, closing one nostril at a time, try to identify the smell of familiar substances such as tobacco or cloves.

5. *Taste*

   Record ability to distinguish sweet, salty solutions. Use solutions of a small amount of sugar and salt dissolved in water, dip cotton tip applicator into solution and apply to client's tongue.

6. *Touch*

   Always perform these tests on opposite, corresponding parts of the body, proceeding with cephalocaudal approach. Compare R/L and periphery with central areas of body. Gently touch skin with wisp of cotton teased from applicator or cotton ball. Client closes eyes and says "yes" or "now" when he feels stimulus. Then ask client to point to area touched.

7. *Temperature*

   Ask client to respond "hot" or "cold" when touched by test tube of warm or cold water. Compare R to L and midline to periphery.

8. *Pain*

Use only a sterile pin! Touch either the point (lightly!) or dull end of safety pin to skin and ask client—eyes closed— to respond, "sharp" or "dull." Compare R to L, midline to periphery.

9. *Stereognosis*

Test client's ability to identify an object through touch by using your finger to write a number on the client's palm and asking him to identify the number; or place a familiar object such as a comb or pen in his hand and ask him to identify it.

10. *Proprioception*

With client's eyes closed, take his index finger and move it up and down. Ask client to say "up" or "down." Repeat with other hand and great toe of each foot.

11. **Vibratory sense*

12. *Sensory environment*

Summarize your own observation (which may or may not agree with what the client or his family reported in the history).

Laboratory Data

Consult client's chart for test results related to sensory status—tonometry (for glaucoma), vision or hearing tests, etc.

Medications

Consult chart and Kardex to determine whether client is on medications that affect sensory status (eye- eardrops, or ointments, for example).

DATE:

ASSESSMENT PRACTICE 38: Initial Plan

Initial Plan

Date: Time: Problem # and name:

S.

O.

A.

P. *Diagnostic:*

Therapeutic:

Teaching:

Referral:

DATE:

ASSESSMENT PRACTICE 39: Progress Note

Progress Note

Date: Time: Problem # and name:

S.

O.

A.

P. *Diagnostic:*

Therapeutic:

Teaching:

Referral:

UNIT 14

Health Status/Discharge Summary

OBJECTIVES

When you have completed this unit, you should be able to:

1. Describe the purposes of a health status/discharge summary.
2. Write a health status/discharge summary of a client with whom you have been working.

PURPOSE OF THE SUMMARY

Sharing the information you have gained about a client's health status and his responses to illness and treatment is vital to continuity of care. The problem-oriented health record system you have been using is a method that helps professionals record in a clearly organized manner the problem-solving process used with each client. There are times, though, when the entire record is too lengthy to serve as an appropriate communications tool between professionals. A *health status summary,* or very brief statement of the most significant data, the problems identified, and the interventions used and their effectiveness, is sometimes more useful. You might present such a health status summary when discussing your client at a conference with professional colleagues, on nursing rounds, or if you terminate with a client and the management of his care will be assumed by others.

If the client is being discharged from a health care facility, or transferred to another facility, a discharge summary is written. A *discharge summary* is problem-oriented and gives a complete, concise summary of each problem and its status at that time. The summary includes subjective and objective data, interventions, progress, client's responses to problems, client and family teaching, and referrals, if any.

WRITING THE SUMMARY

Writing the summary can give you an excellent opportunity to evaluate your total approach to the health problems and needs of the client. Reviewing all the data collected, plans initiated, and interventions attempted should clarify your thinking about how all these are related to the "whole person" who is your client. You may change some priorities or find some not-so-well-coordinated plans for different problems. The health summary is a part of the evaluation step of the problem-solving process and may generate new ideas and new plans.

The discharge summary, like the health status summary, is written in the problem-oriented form. Each problem is identified by its number and name and problems are reviewed in numerical order. This systematic review of problems provides assurance for clients that no problem has been overlooked and provides practitioners with a means of evaluating the care that has been administered.

An example of a discharge summary for a client returning home from a community hospital follows.

7/26/75 2 P.M. Nursing Discharge Note

Mr. Briggs, a 37-year-old married white male, was admitted on 7/20/75 and discharged home on 7/26/75. He will be seeing Dr. Jones for psychotherapy sessions once a week and Mr. Greenstein, nurse practitioner, when needed.

Problems			**Active/Resolved**
7/20/75	#1	Headaches	Active
7/21/75	#2	Myopia	Resolved 7/25/75—new spectacles
7/21/75	#3	Anxiety	Active
7/21/75	#4	Insomnia	Resolved 7/23/75

Problem #1 Headaches

S. Client reported headaches of ↑ frequency from occasional in college, rare for 10 or more years, then weekly to daily for 3 months prior to admission. Describes headaches as dull, constant, pressured "like a band around my head." Unaware of precipitating causes, no trauma, no family history of headaches. Reported headache first day of hospitalization, none since then. At home, used aspirin purchased over the counter, did not always relieve pain.

O. Physical exam and routine lab tests within normal limits: skull x-ray series and EEG negative. Mental status exam revealed anxious, intelligent client with appropriate and cooperative responses to interviewer. Expressed worry about loss of concentration and time at work, and concern over health of his mother, who lives alone in a distant city. Diazepam (Valium) relieved headache in hospital.

A. Objective data shows no organic cause for headaches, which are more typical of emotionally caused tension headaches.

P. Client has agreed to keep daily records of headaches and circumstances when they occur. Medication prescribed—diazepam (Valium). Will call Mr. Greenstein if headaches recur.

Problem #3 Anxiety

S. Client reported difficulty concentrating at work (is an accountant), states "I'm a go-getter, I like to be on top of things." Worried that his mother may need to move in with his family or go to nursing home. Small wt loss and ↓ in appetite in recent weeks.

O. Paced in corridors throughout hospital stay except during visiting hours. Not able to sit for any period of time. Continually asked staff about results of tests.

A. Anxiety, probably related to uncertainty of etiology of headaches, responsibilities to mother, and possible changes in family roles. Was beginning to express some of these concerns in daily talks with primary nurse and in first session with Dr. Jones.

P. Continue to explore with Dr. Jones sources of stress and how to cope with them. Diazepam (Valium) prescribed.

SELECTED BIBLIOGRAPHY

Health Status/Discharge Note

Becknell, Eileen Pearlman, and Dorothy M. Smith: *System of Nursing Practice,* F.A. Davis, Philadelphia, 1975, pp. 117-120.

DATE:

ASSESSMENT PRACTICE 40: Health Status/Discharge Summary

Practice writing a summary now for your client or one of your clients. If you have performed all or most of the assessments with one client, review all your records before writing the summary so that it will reflect the entire problem-solving process.

APPENDIX 1

Additional References

Listed below are additional selected readings and audio-visual materials that can help you expand and implement nursing assessment skills.

Physical Assessment

Alexander, Mary, and Marie Scott Brown: "Physical Examination, Part 4, The Lymphatic System," Nursing '73, **3**:49-59, October 1973.

____, and ____: "Physical Examination, Part 9, Examining the Nose," *Nursing '74,* **4**:35-38, July 1974.

____, and ____: "Physical Examination, Part 14, Examining Male Genitalia," *Nursing '76,* **6**:39-43, February 1976.

____, and ____: "Physical Examination, Part 16, Examining the Musculoskeletal System," *Nursing '76,* **6**:51-56, April 1976.

____, and ____: "Physical Examination, Part 17, Performing the Neurological Examination," *Nursing '76,* **6**:38-43, June 1976.

____, and ____: "Physical Examination, Part 18, Performing the Neurological Examination," *Nursing '76,* **6**:50-55, July 1976.

Brown, Marie Scott, and Mary M. Alexander: 'Physical Examination, Part 15, Examining Female Genitalia," *Nursing '76,* **6**:39-41, March 1976.

Fowler, Marsha D.: "Behold the Right Great Toe," *American Journal of Nursing,* **74**: 1817-1819, 1974.

McFarlane, Judith Medlin: "Pediatric Assessment and Interviewing, Some Simple How-to's for Ambulatory Settings," *Nursing '74,* **4**:66-68, December 1974.

"Patient Assessment: Examination of the Head and Neck," Programmed Instruction, *American Journal of Nursing,* **75,** May 1975.

Physical Assessment Lectures (series of 22 videotape programs), Blue Hill Educational Systems, Spring Valley, N. Y., 1974.

Physical Assessment Examinations (series of 12 videotape programs), Blue Hill Educational Systems, Spring Valley, N. Y., 1975.

Mental and Emotional Assessment

Mental and Emotional Assessment of the Psychiatric Patient (series of 3 videotape programs), Blue Hill Educational Systems, Spring Valley, N. Y., 1975.

APPENDIX 2

Data Collection Outline for Health Status Assessments

CLIENT PROFILE

Source(s) and reliability of data:

Client Profile Name:

Age Sex Birthdate

Ethnicity and place of birth

Occupation

Religious practices

Level of education

Language spoken and ability to read and write

Pattern of socialization and description of friends

Activity-rest pattern: how client spends an average day (be specific)

What are client's current health goals?

FAMILY ASSESSMENT

Client's marital history

With whom does client live now?

Client's position, role in family

Reproductive data (number of pregnancies, living children, contraceptive methods if applicable, menstrual patterns, including menarche and menopause, if applicable)

Availability and use of nonhousehold family members and significant others: relationship with neighbors and other community members

Anything else client views as significant about family

Economic status

Amount and sources of income

Sources of health care payment

Adequacy of economic resources to meet current needs

HOME AND COMMUNITY ASSESSMENT

Living Conditions

Brief description of home by client and/or interviewer: type of dwelling; cooking/eating, bathing, and sleeping arrangements; sanitation—vermin, plumbing, garbage; safety locks, bars at windows; chipping paint and plaster; other factors related to specific health problems such as number of stairs to climb, presence of pets, lighting, ventilation, and screening. Is environment suited to client's health needs? Describe.

Community Assessment

Physical structures in community (high-rise apartments, single-family homes, farm buildings)
Population characteristics (ethnic, age, social class)
Availability and use of community facilities
 Shopping
 Recreation
 Religious
 Social and cultural
 Transportation available to above and to health and social service agencies.

FAMILY STRUCTURE: GENETIC HISTORY

Draw the client's family tree, including that person's generation, parents and grandparents, and children, if any. Under each person's first name, write his or her age or date of death, and any significant health problems known. This would include allergies, alcoholism, obesity, mental illness, arthritis, high blood pressure, heart disease, for example. See the example and code below.

Code

0 = female
□ = male
0—□ = mating
a & w = alive, well
d = died

Example

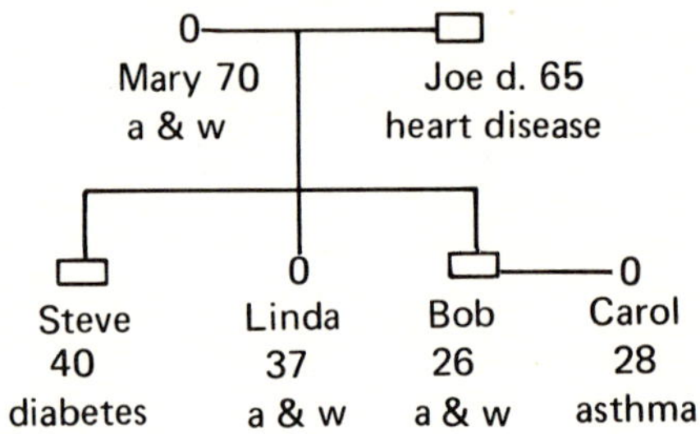

CHIEF COMPLAINT AND HISTORY OF PRESENT PROBLEM

Problem stated in client's own words
Onset
Course
Duration
Character
Aggravating, relieving, associated factors
Treatment and results of treatment

PAST HEALTH HISTORY

Past illnesses (childhood and adulthood)
Accidents
Hospitalizations
Emergency room visits
Travel (outside the country or to areas of known health risk)
Blood transfusions
Allergies

HEALTH MAINTENANCE FLOW SHEET

Utilize interviewing and consultation methods to obtain health maintenance data for your client.

Dates:					Normal Values
Immunizations					
DPT, TOPV, mumps, rubella, influenza, smallpox, etc.					
Tuberculin test					
Chest x ray					
Complete physical examination					
Blood pressure					
EKG					
Dental					
Vision					
Hearing					
Pap smear					
Urinalysis					
WBC with diff					
Hgb					
Hct					
FBS					
Na+					
K+					
Cl^-					
CO_2					
Serology					
Sickle cell trait					

Source: Reprinted with permission of the Herbert H. Lehman College Department of Nursing, Data Base Collection Outline, Problem-Oriented Family Health Record, 1975.

ASSESSMENT OF PHYSICAL STRUCTURE

History

1. Does the client now have or has he ever had in the past:
   a. skin changes (rashes, lesions, infections, any other changes)
   b. nail changes (breaking, brittle, color change)
   c. hair changes
   d. bone fracture
   e. swelling or other change in body part
   f. loss or deformity of body part
2. Does the client use any prostheses (dentures, artificial limb) or supportive devices such as cane, crutches, built-up shoe?
3. Client's usual hygiene habits (bathing, brushing teeth, hair care, nail care).
4. Client's knowledge of hygiene needs (your evaluation based on information in (3) above).
5. Is the client using any medications for his skin (soaps, ointments), or any medications in relation to any problems he has stated? Include summary of client's understanding of medications.

Physical Examination

1. *Statement of General Appearance*
   Briefly describe client by shape/build, size/proportions, symmetry of body parts, apparent age, and/or a few other phrases which would distinguish him from others in a waiting room.
2. *Skin and Hair*
   You can examine skin and hair as you proceed in cephalocaudal manner to assess body structures. For example, as you examine the head, you would assess the skin of the face and scalp, and note hair condition and distribution. What to check for in skin assessment: color, lesions, scars, birthmarks, cleanliness, texture, turgor, temperature, wetness-dryness, intactness. Remember to include a skin assessment in each area of the physical structure assessment.
3. *Head*
   a. shape/proportion
   b. irregularities or asymmetry of face and skull
   c. hair color, distribution, texture
   d. skin
4. *Eyes*
   a. eyebrows present
   b. eyelids (drooping, lashes present)
   c. conjunctiva (color)
   d. sclerae (color)
   e. iris (color)
   f. pupils (color, shape, equality)
5. *Ears*
   a. symmetry
   b. presence of wax, discharge
6. *Nose*
   a. shape, symmetry on face
   b. discharge
7. *Mouth*
   a. symmetry
   b. color of lips, condition
   c. tongue (color, hydration)
   d. teeth (condition, hygiene)

e. gums (color, condition)
f. buccal mucosa (hydration, color)

8. *Neck*
    a. symmetry
    b. skin
9. *Chest*
    a. deformities of thorax (barrel-shaped chest, "pigeon" breast)
    b. skin
10. *Breasts*
    a. development (relative to age)
    b. symmetry, shape
    c. nipple discharge
    d. skin
11. *Back*
    a. contour (deformities such as kyphosis, scoliosis)
    b. skin
12. *Abdomen*
    a. contour (protuberant, flat)
    b. scars
    c. skin
13. *Genitalia, male*
    Note developmental status, skin and hair, any swelling or discharge of:
    a. penis
    b. urethra
    c. scrotum
    d. rectum
14. *Genitalia, female*
    Note developmental status, skin and hair, any swelling or discharge of:
    a. labia majora and minora
    b. urethra
    c. vaginal opening
    d. rectum
15. *Extremities*
    arms and hands
    a. symmetry
    b. joint swelling
    c. skin
    d. nails (color, shape, mobility)
    legs and feet
    a. symmetry
    b. varicosities
    c. joint swelling
    d. skin
    e. nails

Laboratory Data

Any x-ray reports indicating normal or abnormal structures (such as enlarged heart, healed fracture)

Medications Related to Physical Structure

Check chart, Kardex, physician's order sheet to validate client's report. Include generic and brand names of drug, dose, route of administration, when given.[1]

ASSESSMENT OF MOBILITY/COMFORT/REST

History

1. *Mobility—Client's perception of the following:*
   a. Are there any medical restrictions on activity (physician's prescription for bed rest, bathroom privileges, etc.)?
   b. Are there any institutional restrictions on activity (when are visitors allowed, does the client need a pass if he wishes to go out for a few hours, are bedrails, restraints, used)?
   c. Are there any environmental restrictions on activity (what is available for physical exercise and activities, and what intellectual stimulation is available)?
   d. Does the client now have, or has he ever had in the past:
      (1) paralysis
      (2) weakness
      (3) contractures
      (4) abnormal movements (spasms, tremors, tics)
      (5) stiffness
      (6) trauma (accidents, injuries)
      (7) swelling, pain, or tenderness
      (8) difficulty with walking, reaching, or other movements
   e. Any aids used for ambulation (cane, crutches, chair, walker, etc.)?
   f. Medications client is taking to aid mobility/activity. Include summary of client's understanding of medications.

How does the client describe the following?

2. *Sleep*
   a. Normal sleep pattern (number of hours, time, whether the client feels rested, naps).
   b. Any changes in sleep pattern—describe.
   c. Characteristics of sleep (sound, light, dreams, nightmares, restless, quiet).
   d. Aids used for sleep (beverages, positional comfort, reading, rituals, medications—sedatives, hypnotics).
3. *Comfort*
   a. Presence of pain or discomfort (onset, progression, duration, character, location, course, aggravating or relieving factors).
   b. Treatment to relieve pain or discomfort (prior to and during current experience—analgesics, positioning, exercise, compresses, talking about it).

Physical Examination

1. *Mobility*
   a. general movements (smooth, jerky, tremor)
   b. handedness
   c. range of joint motion (evaluate and record on chart on page 179)
   d. ability to perform activities of daily living (evaluate and record on chart on page 180)

[1] Beginning students may want to include expected effects of the drug.

Assessment of Range of Joint Motion

First determine which motions can be performed actively without assistance by the client, then assess passive range of motion for joints which cannot be moved through the full normal range actively.

F = full motion; P = partial motion; 0 = no motion

Specify motion in degrees if possible.

Joints	Motions	Observed Motions			
		Active		Passive	
Neck	flexion				
	extension				
	rotation				
Trunk	flexion				
	extension				
		Right	Left	Right	Left
Shoulder	flexion				
	extension				
	abduction				
	adduction				
	int. rotation				
	ext. rotation				
Elbow	flexion				
	suppination				
	pronation				
Wrist	flexion				
	extension				
	ul. deviation				
	ra. deviation				
Fingers	flexion				
	extension				
Thumb	flexion				
	extension				
Hip	flexion				
	extension				
	abduction				
	adduction				
	int. rotation				
	ext. rotation				
Knee	flexion				
	extension				
Ankle	flexion				
	extension				
	inversion				
	eversion				
Toes	flexion				
	extension				

Assessment for Activities of Daily Living

Grade only activities actually observed as follows:

G = good, independent and at least fairly efficient
F = fair, very slow, insecure, or tiring
P = partial, requires supervision or some assistance
O = zero, not even partial performance possible

Hygiene		**Locomotion**	
Brush, comb hair		Chair, sitting down	
Brush teeth		Chair, getting up	
Wash hands		Room walking	
Wash face		Stairs up	
Wash feet		Stairs down	
Turn faucet		Walk, turn corner	
Take shower		Walk to bathroom	
Take bath (tub)		Get into car	
Use handkerchief			
Eating		**Writing, Reading**	
Eat with Spoon		Write by hand	
Eat with fork		Use typewriter	
Use knife		Unfold newspaper	
Butter bread		Hold book	
Drink-glass, cup		Turn pages	
Dressing		**Miscellaneous**	
Undershirt, bra		Doorknob	
Shorts, panties		Use drawer	
Shirt, blouse		Dial telephone	
Trousers, skirt		Use scissors	
Socks, stockings		Use keys	
Slip on Shoes		Move chair	
Tie laces		Count coins	
Jacket, dress			
Zipper, buttons			

Source: Adapted from and used with permission of Armour Pharmaceuticals, "Evaluation Chart: Activities of Daily Living."

e. stance
   (1) posture when standing
   (2) need for support when standing (equilibrium—balance)
f. gait
   (1) assistance needed for ambulation
   (2) posture when walking
   (3) observe for shuffling, limping, foot dragging, foot slapping, if arms swing freely

2. *Sleep*

   As suggested earlier, if you are not present when client is sleeping, you may want to confer with family and/or staff members regarding client's sleep patterns, including naps. The Kardex and nurses' notes on the chart may also have information regarding sleep patterns.

3. *Comfort*

   Indications of possible pain or discomfort

   a. restlessness, withdrawal, difficulty in sleeping, loss of appetite
   b. increase in muscle tension
   c. changes in physical structure (swelling, skin intactness—color—texture, trauma)
   d. change in temperature, BP, respirations (see oxygenation assessment)

Laboratory Data

Include x-ray reports indicating joint abnormalities, bone deformities, fractures.

Medications Related to Mobility/Comfort/Rest

Such medications include stimulants, skeletal muscle relaxants, analgesics, tranquilizers. Include the same data for reviewing medications pertaining to mobility as you utilized in reviewing medications in the physical structure assessment.

OXYGENATION ASSESSMENT

History

1. *Respiratory*

   a. Does the client now have, or has he ever had in the past:
      chest pain
      cough (productive, chronic, acute, time of day, with activity)
      expectoration (color, amount, odor, viscosity, hemoptysis)
      dyspnea
      orthopnea
      frequent colds
   b. Does the client use any supportive devices for breathing (nebulizer, humidifier, respirator)?
   c. Does the client use any medications that affect respiratory status?
   d. What are the client's impressions of impairment and limitations, if any, of respiratory status on daily life (activities, sleep, habits)?
   e. If client experiences anxiety or apprehension, does he see this as affecting breathing? If so, describe.

2. *Circulatory*

   a. Does the client now have, or has he ever had in the past:
      heart disease
      chest or epigastric pain
      palpitation
      fatigue
      heart murmur
      problems with blood pressure
      cyanosis
      edema
      cold extremities
      pains in legs when walking
      anemia
      bruising

   b. What are the client's impressions of impairment and limitations, if any, of circulatory status on daily life (sleep, activities, habits)?

   c. Is the client taking any medications that affect circulatory status?

3. *Temperature status*

   Give client's description of:

   a. feelings of warmth and cold
   b. usual measures for temperature comfort
   c. perspiration (presence, absence, pattern, night sweats)
   d. environmental temperature and humidity
   e. use of medications that affect temperature status

Physical Examination

1. *Head*	Rate	Quality	Rhythm
a. R temporal pulse			
L temporal pulse			
b. eyes	R		L
(1) sclera (color)			
(2) conjunctiva (color)			
c. nose			
(1) deviation			
(2) breathing through nose			
d. mouth			
(1) color of lips, mucous membrane			
(2) patency of airway (clear, obstructed)			

2. *Neck*	Rate	Quality	Rhythm
a. R carotid pulse			
b. L carotid pulse			

3. *Chest*

   a. size and shape (ratio of anteroposterior diameter to lateral diameter)

   b. respirations

      (1) rate, rhythm, depth, ease, noise
      (2) change in relation to activity level, position, emotion, pain, humidity, air pollution
      (3) ventilatory motion (abdominal, thoracic)
      (4) sternal retractions
      (5) cough, wheezing

4. *Apical impulse*	Rate	Quality	Rhythm

5. *Back (contour and postural influences on respiration—kyphosis, lordosis)*
6. *Arms* Rate Quality Rhythm
   a. R brachial pulse
   b. L brachial pulse
   c. R radial pulse
   d. L radial pulse
   e. pulse deficit (apical rate—radial rate)
   f. pulse response in relation to activity level, anxiety, pain
   g. skin temperature, color
   h. nails
      (1) color
      (2) clubbing
   i. blood pressure Systolic/muffling/diastolic
      (1) R arm sitting
      (2) L arm sitting
      (3) R arm lying
      (4) L arm lying
      (5) Pulse pressure
7. *Buttocks (sacral edema)*
8. *Legs*
   a. skin color, temperature
   b. pulses Rate Quality Rhythm
      (1) R femoral
      (2) L femoral
      (3) R popliteal
      (4) L popliteal
      (5) R dorsalis pedis
      (6) L dorsalis pedis
      (7) R posterior tibial
      (8) L posterior tibial
   c. edema (extent, location)
9. *Body temperature (measure with thermometer)*
   a. oral
   b. rectal
   c. axillary
10. *Exercise tolerance (changes in vital signs, amount of activity tolerated)*

Laboratory Data[2]

1. Respiratory-chest x ray, skin test, blood gas analysis—PO_2, PCO_2, blood pH.
2. Circulatory-chest x ray, hemoglobin, hematocrit

Medications Related to Respiratory, Circulatory, Temperature Status

1. A classification of medications affecting respiratory status includes bronchodilators, antibiotics, antitussives, expectorants, nasal decongestants.
2. A classification of medications affecting circulatory status includes vasodilators, antihypertensives, vasoconstrictors, cardiac glycosides, antianemic drugs, anticoagulent drugs, and antiarrhythmic drugs.
3. A classification of medication affecting temperature status includes an antipyretic.

[2]Some of these values may be entered on the Health Maintenance Flow Sheet.

NUTRITION/ELIMINATION ASSESSMENT

History

1. *Nutrition*
   a. appetite
   b. usual eating patterns and usual times (use chart on page 185)
   c. eating behavior (gulper, nibbler, eat-and-run, fast-and-feast)
   d. food likes and dislikes
   e. food restrictions (culture, religion, allergies, food intolerance—describe)
   f. changes in pattern (special diet, appetite changes, stress)
   g. assistance needed in eating
   h. diet supplements (preparations such as sustagen, vitamins)
   i. weight gain or loss (steady, sporadic, over what period of time)
   j. symbolic meaning of food (socialization, love, reward, eat when nervous)
   k. past or present experiences of
      (1) diabetes
      (2) nutritional disease
      (3) flatulence
      (4) burping
      (5) nausea, vomiting
      (6) heartburn
      (7) pain
      (8) difficulty in swallowing, tasting
   l. artificial means of food intake (tube feeding, hyperalimentation)
   m. usual care of teeth (daily, dentist's visits; if dentures, type, fit, effectiveness)
   n. use of any medications affecting metabolism, digestion of foods, nutritional status
2. *Fluid balance*
   a. pattern of fluid intake (amount in 24 h, types preferred)
   b. changes in fluid intake (related to health problem, increase or decrease)
   c. past or present experiences of
      (1) thirst
      (2) weight gain or loss
      (3) edema
      (4) neuromuscular weakness or irritability
3. *Pattern of fluid elimination*
   a. sweating (times, amount)
   b. urination (frequency, urgency, pain, burning, dribbling, nocturia)
   c. urine (amount, color, odor, unusual constituents)
   d. method of elimination (toilet, bedpan, commode, urinal, needs assistance)
   e. continence/incontinence (circumstances, ways of coping)
   f. changes in usual pattern—describe
   g. drainage from wounds
   h. use of any medication affecting fluid balance and/or elimination

24-HOUR NUTRITION SUMMARY

For each meal and/or snack, record the food, its amount, and how it was prepared, under the appropriate column. A peanut butter and jelly sandwich, for example, might be recorded as 2 slices white bread under the "bread and cereals" column, 2 tablespoons peanut butter and 1 tablespoon jelly under the condiments column along with the time and place where it was consumed. Another example would be a broiled chicken leg prepared without salt eaten at 5 p.m. at the hospital cafeteria recorded under the "meats, fish, and poultry" column.

Meal or Snack	Meats, Fish and Poultry	Fruits and Vegetables	Milk and Dairy Products	Bread and Cereals	**Other** (condiments such as salt, salad dressing, gravy; soft drinks and alcoholic beverages, etc.)
Breakfast Time ______ Place ______					
Lunch Time ______ Place ______					
Dinner Time ______ Place ______					
Other (Snacks, Supplements) Time ______ Place ______					
	Evaluation of Adequacy: Evaluate the nutritional adequacy of your client's food intake in each of the above categories, using the "basic four" requirements.				

4. *Pattern of bowel elimination*
    a. usual pattern (frequency, time of day, aids normally used—beverages, exercises, enemas)
    b. character of stool (color, amount, odor, consistency, unusual constituents)
    c. diarrhea, constipation (acute, chronic)
    d. continence/incontinence (circumstances, ways of coping)
    e. changes in usual pattern—describe
    f. hemorrhoids
    g. artificial orifices for elimination (ileal conduit—urine, colostomy—bowel, client's way of caring for this)

Physical Examination[3]

1. *Height and weight (metric system)*
2. *Head*
    a. level of consciousness
    b. hair (texture, sheen, distribution)
    c. skin (texture, dryness, turgor)
    d. mouth
        (1) mucous membranes (intactness, dry, moist, color, presence of debris, crusts, lesions)
        (2) breath
        (3) teeth (dentulous, edentulous, condition)
        (4) gums (color, condition)
        (5) tongue (dry, presence of crust, debris)
3. *Throat*
    a. exudate, injection
    b. ability to swallow
4. *Abdomen*
    a. contour
    b. bowel sounds
5. *Rectum*
    a. hemorrhoids
    b. fissures
6. *Arms and hands*
    a. skin (texture, dryness, turgor)
    b. ability to feed self
7. *Legs and feet*
    a. skin (texture, dryness, turgor)
    b. edema (pattern and location, extent)
8. *Intake and output*

    Obtain a 24-hour record of your client's I & O and record, using metric liquid measure. Your client, if able, may help you by keeping a record of this. Evaluate I & O in terms of adequacy and meeting client's needs.
9. *Urine*

    color, clear or cloudy, odor, unusual constituents—compare with normal values
10. *Stool*

    color, form, odor, consistency, unusual constituents—compare with normal values

[3]*Note:* If you have already recorded this data in previous assessments, refer to those assessments rather than repeating descriptions here.

Laboratory Data

1. *Electrolytes*[4] — Normal values
2. *Blood sugar*[4] — Normal values
3. *Urine*[4] — Normal values
   a. color
   b. pH
   c. specific gravity
   d. sugar and acetone
   e. WBC
4. *Stool* — Normal values
   a. eggs/parasites
   b. occult blood

Medications Related to Nutrition/Elimination/Fluid Balance

(Objective data—from Kardex, chart, M.D.'s order sheet)

1. A classification of medications affecting metabolism and digestion of foods and nutritional status includes minerals, vitamins, hormones, antacids, antiemetics.
2. A classification of medications affecting fluid balance and elimination includes diuretics, hormones, drugs acting on bladder, urinary antiseptics.
3. A classification of medications affecting bowel elimination includes cathartics, antidiarrheics, stool softeners.

MENTAL/EMOTIONAL STATUS ASSESSMENT

History

1. Client's perception and understanding of his health problem(s) and goals of medical and nursing therapy.
2. Beliefs and attitudes about illness (sickness as punishment).
3. Previous experience with, and reaction to, illness and/or hospitalization.
4. Client's description of himself; how does he see himself as a person?
   a. general mood and emotional responses
   b. role played or assigned in family, community
   c. concept of self (sense of worth, self-esteem)
   d. reactions to stress and ways of coping with stressful situations
   e. patterns of relating to others
   f. sexuality
      (1) sexual preference (homosexual/heterosexual)
      (2) pleasure/discomfort
      (3) responsiveness
   g. special concerns or fears
5. Client's perception of reality orientation—time, place, month, year.
6. Client's perception of memory—remote and recent.
7. Has client ever had any wish to die or to harm anyone else? Has anyone in his family attempted suicide or violent behavior?
   a. History of attempts, plans, intent to carry out plan.
   b. Has client experienced a recent loss? Are there other provoking factors?

[4] Some of these values may be entered on the Health Maintenance Flow Sheet.

8. Has client sensed changes in behavior, perception, thought process, mood, anxiety, body functioning, or changes in any of the above areas?
9. Is client using any substances that alter his emotional responses? (Include prescribed drugs, tranquilizers, sedatives, antidepressants, amphetamines; "street" drugs such as marijuana, LSD; over-the-counter drugs; alcoholic beverages; coffee, tea, and cola beverages containing caffeine.)

Examination

1. *Overall impression*
   Briefly write your general impression of your client, including apparent physical condition, general health, approximate height and weight, posture, eye contact, appropriateness of dress for age-sex-season-setting, and relatedness to you as the interviewer.
2. *Degree of reality orientation*
   a. knowledge of time-place-month-year
   b. memory—remote and recent
3. *Intellectual development relative to age*
   Estimate normal, above- or below-average intelligence, mental retardation.
4. *Behavior*
   a. motor activity (unusual movements, over- or under-active)
   b. awareness of environment
5. *Speech*
   a. sound (loud, soft, monotonic)
   b. rate
6. *Emotional expression (mood or affect)*
   a. appropriateness to topic being discussed
   b. overall impression of mood/affect
7. *Thought processes*
   a. quality of responses—appropriate or inappropriate
   b. ability to understand and follow directions
   c. attention span; connections between ideas
   d. spontaneity, flexibility/rigidity
8. *Thought content*
   a. central themes (what client talks about)
   b. special preoccupations (hallucinations, delusions, phobias, obsessive thoughts, compulsive behaviors)
9. *Ways of coping with stressful situations*
   use of defense mechanisms, "fight or flight"
10. *Ego strengths*
    a. judgment (how to budget money, plan activities, dress appropriately)
    b. sense of reality of world and self (realistic perception of self and environment)
    c. regulation and control of drives and impulses (pattern of planned versus impulsive behavior)
    d. ability to relate to others
    e. functional abilities, such as in work, school, homemaking, parenting

Laboratory Data

1. EEG findings
2. Consider also normal and abnormal findings from other assessment areas since mental/emotional status affects and is affected by physical health.

Medications That Affect Mental/Emotional Status

1. A classification of medications affecting mental/emotional status includes major and minor tranquilizers, antidepressants, hallucinogenic drugs, sedatives, and amphetamines.

SENSORY ASSESSMENT

This assessment is part of a complete neurological assessment, which involves evaluation of motor functioning and perceptual abilities as well as sensory assessment. In the sensory assessment outline which follows, the starred items indicate additional data which would be included in a more complete neurological examination. Data listed under other assessments in this workbook are also collected in a complete neurological examination, for example, data on gait, balance, involuntary motions, level of consciousness, ability to swallow, symmetry of eyelids.

History

Enter dates for previous vision and hearing testing on Health Maintenance Flow Sheet.

1. *Eyes*
   a. how client evaluates own vision
   b. corrective lenses used
   c. any known vision problems
   d. extent to which problems interfere with ADL
   e. diplopia, blurring, photophobia, color blindness, squinting, strabismus
   f. pain
   g. any other eye problems or recent changes in any of the above
2. *Ears*
   a. how client evaluates own hearing
   b. infections, dizziness, tinnitis, pain
   c. known hearing problems
   d. extent to which problems interfere with ADL
   e. use of hearing aid, ability to lipread, or other ways of compensating for loss
   f. any other ear problems or recent changes in any of the above
3. *Nose*
   a. client's evaluation of sense of smell
   b. any known problems, such as nosebleeds, sinus problems, hayfever
4. *Mouth*
   a. client's evaluation of sense of taste
   b. review Nutrition/Elimination Assessment for additional relevant data
5. *Touch*
   a. ability to feel heat, cold, pain, vibration, movement, touch on all body parts
   b. any other problems of touch (paresthesias, heightened sensitivity to touch)
6. *Sensory environment*
   Note client's description of quality and quantity and appropriateness of environmental stimuli. What is client's preferred level of environmental stimulation (high, moderate, low)?

Examination

1. *Eyes*
   a. visual acuity (use Snellen chart)
      R eye
      L eye
      both eyes
   b. pupils R L
      pupils equal?
      pupils round?
      response to light
      response to accommodation
      *extraocular movements, visual fields

2. *Ears* R L

   a. hears ticking watch (at what distance)

   b. hears spoken voice (at what distance)

   c. hears whispered voice (at what distance)

   d. *Weber test

      *Rinne test

3. *Speech*

   a. Evaluate conversational speech for fluency, hesitation, pronunciation. If any difficulty is suspected, test client's ability to repeat words, phrases, sentences; ask client to name two or three common objects (comb, watch, pencil).

   b. Record client's ability to follow simple directions (squeeze my hand, give me the pencil). If client has difficulty following spoken directions, try using gestures or written words.

4. *Smell*

   Beginning-level examinations usually do not include testing smell. If a problem is reported in the history, you could perform a simple test by asking client to close his eyes and, closing one nostril at a time, try to identify the smell of familiar substances such as tobacco or cloves.

5. *Taste*

   Record ability to distinguish sweet, salty solutions. Use solutions of a small amount of sugar and salt dissolved in water, dip cotton tip applicator into solution and apply to client's tongue.

6. *Touch*

   Always perform these tests on opposite, corresponding parts of the body, proceeding with cephalocaudal approach. Compare R/L and periphery with central areas of body. Gently touch skin with wisp of cotton teased from applicator or cotton ball. Client closes eyes and says "yes" or "now" when he feels stimulus. Then ask client to point to area touched.

7. *Temperature*

   Ask client to respond "hot" or "cold" when touched by test tube of warm or cold water. Compare R to L and midline to periphery.

8. *Pain*

   Use only a sterile pin! Touch either the point (lightly!) or dull end of safety pin to skin and ask client—eyes closed—to respond, "sharp" or "dull." Compare R to L, midline to periphery.

9. *Stereognosis*

   Test client's ability to identify an object through touch by using your finger to write a number on the client's palm and ask him to identify the number; or place a familiar object such as a comb or pen in his hand and ask him to identify it.

10. *Proprioception*

    With client's eyes closed, take his index finger and move it up and down. Ask client to say "up" or "down." Repeat with other hand and great toe of each foot.

11. **Vibratory sense*

12. *Sensory environment*

    Summarize your own observations (which may or may not agree with what the client or his family reported in the history).

Laboratory Data

Consult client's chart for test results related to sensory status—tonometry (for glaucoma), vision or hearing tests, etc.

Medications

Consult chart and Kardex to determine whether client is on medications that affect sensory status (eye- eardrops, or ointments, for example).